Body
Intelligence

by the same author

You Are How You Move
Experiential Chi Kung
ISBN 978 1 84819 014 6

of related interest

Meet Your Body
CORE Bodywork and Rolfing Tools to Release
Bodymindcore Trauma
Noah Karrasch
ISBN 978 1 84819 016 0

The Insightful Body
Healing with SomaCentric Dialoguing
Julie McKay
ISBN 978 1 84819 030 6

Curves, Twists and Bends
A Practical Guide to Pilates for Scoliosis
Annette Wellings with Alan Herdman
ISBN 978 1 84819 025 2

Body
Intelligence

Creating a New Environment

Second Edition

Ged Sumner

Singing Dragon
London and Philadelphia

First published in 2006
by Ged Sumner

This second enlarged edition published in 2010
by Singing Dragon
an imprint of Jessica Kingsley Publishers
116 Pentonville Road
London N1 9JB, UK
and
400 Market Street, Suite 400
Philadelphia, PA 19106, USA

www.singing-dragon.com

Copyright © Ged Sumner 2006 and 2010

Library of Congress Cataloging in Publication Data
A CIP catalog record for this book is available from the Library of Congress

British Library Cataloguing in Publication Data
A CIP catalogue record for this book is available from the British Library

ISBN 978 1 84819 026 9

Printed and bound in the United States by
Thomson-Shore, 7300 W. Joy Road, Dexter, MI 48130

Contents

Preface

At eight years old I believed I was Mr Spock, and as a result continuously performed the Vulcan mind grip on my younger sister. Despite my eager persistence I never managed to experience the melding of minds and, looking back, my sister was really very generous about it. Curiously, some 20 years later I became a craniosacral therapist and started to understand some of the experiences that Mr Spock was having. At last my persistence had paid off, although my blood never went green and my ears, I can assure you, are not pointy. In fact, I found myself having access to a remarkable therapy that brought me into a very special and highly sensitive relationship with my body and educated me into how the body naturally adjusts itself and has an intelligence all of its own – something nobody had ever told me before.

As life continued it seemed like I was missing out on something mysterious, yet hugely significant. Despite the arrogance of my teenage years, I soon realized how little I knew and wondered, like many others, whether there was a deeper intelligence/force in our lives. I was particularly astonished to find how little I knew about the body. For instance, when people spoke of their 'stomach' I realized I didn't really know what they meant exactly. I knew they weren't referring to their real, actual stomach, because their hands were indicating their abdomen (although at the time I didn't even know that word!). How many times have you placed your hands on your gut and called it your stomach? So, like many others, I just didn't know the detail of what was in my abdomen, which, when you think about it, is kind of crazy, because I was using and experiencing it every day. I became determined to know how it all works and so, over a period of many years, I consumed anatomy and physiology books and atlases of the human body, becoming even more fascinated by the deeper meaning of the body, looking at its form and function, and getting to know it in a deeper and more holistic way, which led to surprising revelations.

In my mid twenties, I developed a strong interest in Chi Kung and other Eastern spiritual traditions. Chi Kung remains a total inspiration. It enables me to feel 'chi', or 'vital energy' – something you cannot see or measure through the body. The best way to experience 'chi' is by being in tune with your body through posture, breathing, awareness and movement. The more connected you are, the more you feel it – and it's available all the time. This helped me to deepen my interest in my own internal states, continuously refining my skills, and I started to wonder about consciousness, thoughts, emotions and the body and how they all intertwine. This led to me retreating from the world for several years to lead a meditative life doing spiritual practice and reading about mysticism, religion and philosophy: in particular, about the life of saints and mystics and their discoveries about man's inner nature. I began to understand that the body is the gateway to a subtler universe within us that permeates throughout everything. My interest in the Tao sprang from this time, along with a comprehension of a universal natural intelligence moving around and within us that orders things, and with which you can become more coherent through stillness and listening to your body.

I went on to study shiatsu and healing, which helped me to get a view into energy and the body. I learnt how we can heal ourselves through a healthy and conscious lifestyle, making right choices that lead to an empowered life, and also how the mind, body and emotions are inseparable, contrary to how they are often depicted.

Throughout this time I had been interested in the work of Freud and how he defined the unconscious and its connection to the body's biological drives. I became equally fascinated with Jung's idea of a universal mind. Curious about how the mind functions, I went on to study attachment therapy – a form of psychotherapy that looks at the way we relate to our care givers in the first couple of years of life. It states that relationship is critical for our physical development and mental well-being and that these first relationships are the most important experiences we have. They create the foundations for how we view ourselves for the rest of our lives. Ironically, it was through exploring attachment theory that I really began to understand how the body, even more than the mind, is the receptacle for all our experiences, from our pre-verbal states right through adulthood. I finally understood, more than ever, that the key to unlocking and transforming our past lies in finding new relationships to our own bodies.

Having traversed the paths of both self-taught and formal education, I now view things differently, perhaps more freely. Having gained a thorough theoretical understanding of our body mechanics, my self-taught inner explorations allowed me to discover the body in a more intuitive and natural way, much like looking at a work of art and allowing oneself to be impressed by an inner meaning that goes beyond the form.

It is with this combination of experience that I wrote this book, to share my learnings over the years and to give you an opportunity to discover yourself in your own unique and individual way. I have, therefore, deliberately given information in a way that is easily accessible without being rigid and imposing. The truth, in the end, will lie within your own sense of yourself and this, too, will change as time moves on. This book has been written to help you connect, in an easy and open manner, to the wealth of vital information and experience that lies just beneath your skin.

Know Your Body

This book will introduce you to new ideas of how your body works and will, I hope, lead you to an enriched sense of self.

The anatomy of your body will be explored without the complexity of medical terminology and, in its place, common descriptions will be used to allow you to envisage the different and complicated levels of your human body. This will change your perception of the body you live in, showing you the way to higher levels of health and bodily intelligence that are naturally yours and accessible all the time. The book will explore the difference between being in a sensitive relationship with our bodies and being, essentially, numb to the world. What would be the benefit to us, the environment, family, friends and, in the broader context, our world, if we were more sensitive? What does this mean? In this context, it literally means having a capacity to perceive our bodies via the sense organs, in as deep a manner as possible, and then to be able to receive impulses/information from the environment. This new-found sensitivity would work its way into all areas of our lives: in our relationships, in how we look after ourselves and how we experience the world around us – putting all that we do into perspective, and recognizing the amount of stress we subject our bodies to without realizing.

When you think about it, how do we get through life without knowing about our body? Really, what else is there to know? It's so much of who we are, perhaps all of who we are. We experience the world through our body senses: we move, we eat, we touch, breathe and talk, responding to our environment through our body. But most people don't know how their body works or what it's composed of. Even though there has been a 'quantum leap' in medical science over the past 40 years, revealing so much about the mysteries of the human body, from its functioning at a systemic level right down to genetic and molecular levels, people still know very little. Perhaps it takes time for new knowledge to enter the general consciousness and therefore start to change our day-to-day lives. We are taught biology at school as just another subject, something you can elect to take or not, when really there's only one necessary subject – the vital subject of the body. Young people are introduced to biology and the science of the body with an air of incredulousness. Academic styles of teaching make it hard to see the information as human, so it is difficult to relate to it within the context of your own body and your life. No wonder lots of us are body unaware and often living in a mental space disconnected from our bodies. We are not educated in a way that links the scientific knowledge of the body to how we experience ourselves, and also the environment, through our bodies.

At the same time, we are subject to ideas about our body, mostly through the media, on a continual basis. This has never before been such a powerful force as it is today. The perpetual images of the 'perfect body' and ideas of what it means to be healthy create many different, and often conflicting, feelings about our bodies and how they function. This has an effect on our body image and, therefore, on our sense of self. It is vital to explore these ideas, to understand their origins and know how they affect us, so that we can begin to disentangle ourselves from a false image and move into a more authentic relationship with our body. They are strong forces that can reduce our possibilities in life and transforming them can lead to more creative ways of living.

With so much information bombarding us, it is therefore imperative that we do take the time to connect with our bodies. Often illness and poor health stems from the lack of awareness and connection. Interestingly, it is often the case that people get ill when they retire or go on holiday, as it's only then that they have time to let their bodies rest and be listened to. The ramifications of poor body awareness are enormous; when we are disconnected from our body we are disconnected from our feelings, from relationships with others and from our environment. The benefits that good body awareness could have for the individual, for society and for nature are therefore huge: imagine a world full of empathetic human beings.

The more sensitive you become to your body the more you start to hear its needs. Then you naturally want to feed it healthy food and offer it intelligent exercise, not abuse it or exhaust it. You start to move into a harmonious relationship with your body and everything about you will change. Being in harmony with your body is the start of being in harmony with yourself and who you are and how you want to lead your life.

This book is an attempt to make the body, your body, more accessible. There are millions of facts about the body from modern medical science that aren't necessary for you to know in order to grasp the basics of how your body works. Instead, certain facts are presented here that highlight key qualities and functions of the body, derived from a mixture of Western medical science, Eastern concepts of health and medicine, and alternative body therapy approaches. Most of the medical 'lingo' has been purposefully expelled, to make it more reader-friendly, keeping only the more commonly used terms that may be useful to know, and this in itself might help to break down the negative reactions towards medical terminology.

As well as learning about the mechanics of your body, you will be guided through some practical exercises. This is an attempt to bring your awareness into relationship with the felt sense of any particular area we may be discussing and you will gain much information from this experience. Setting up the space for these exercises is important. It's best to be in a quiet space, away from other people and phones, so that you won't be disturbed. Try to find the best place in your house for doing this. It's probably best to sit while you are doing the exercises – find a chair that's comfortable and upright so that you can experience gravity and your spine and posture can be aligned. You can also do the exercises standing up – just make sure your feet are wide enough apart so that you feel stable. You could try them lying down too, but make sure you don't start to feel soporific as you may doze off!

As you move through the exercises, you may notice that it's a struggle to feel certain body structures or functions whilst others you can relate to easily. You will be encouraged to pay particular attention to this, as it will indicate where you orientate to most in your body. You might not be as connected to certain tissues or parts of your body as others and this is quite a common experience. In this way you can start to construct a 'body map' that will show your body awareness in detail. From this, new gateways of awareness will open as you start to recognize all of your body and listen to the detail of what's going on. Much of this will be wonderful, but some of it might bring up difficult feelings as you start to make connections with your body memory: the body is a memory bank of all your experiences. Our bodies hold the landscape of the many events in our lives; some of the landscape will no doubt have turbulent weather, which may contain difficult feelings that are unresolved. Remember, the emphasis of the exercises is to open up to an underlying order that will bring about integration of body physiology with your thoughts and feelings.

When identifying the state of your body, something wonderful happens – an automatic process of change begins. Just becoming aware of something brings about change, in order to better accommodate 'something new'. That new something could be as simple as a new state of being and it can lead to a whole lot more. As your body awareness increases through the exercises, you will notice physical changes occurring: your body will, literally, re-posture itself, there will be reorganization of structures around each other, a re-alignment that brings about a new physiology; all of which will often be followed by mental or emotional shifts. You therefore begin to feel different, move differently and think differently. This process will affect all parts of your body, and by using the exercises for the particular areas of the body that you have difficulty relating to, you will bring about deep change to your whole body. This will happen over time with repetition of the exercises. All of this leads to a rare and precious state: 'Integrated Body Awareness' – a state of relating to the whole of your body in the present. This naturally creates greater vitality and clarity of mind.

HOW TO USE THIS BOOK

Initially it's advisable to read through the whole book to get a sense of it and attempt some of the exercises. Each chapter contains a lot of information and you may discover new ways of perceiving and understanding that will take time to digest. The information and concepts presented in this book cannot be understood by the intellect alone. Much of the material is concerned with how things relate to each other and their deeper meanings. The exercises themselves will take time to become familiar and time to assimilate. Therefore you need to consider that the chapters are things to keep working with. The order of the chapters is such that the more obviously familiar things, such as bones and joints, are dealt with in the beginning and the least familiar later on. However, this may not work for you as an individual. It may be that you relate more strongly to the material in the chapter on the brain than the one on joints, in which case, perhaps that's revealing something about yourself, and staying with the brain exercises first may unveil the rest of you more clearly. The other consideration may be that you need to spend time with the joint exercises and contemplate the ideas explored within them to make them more accessible. Perhaps a combination of both would work over time.

If you are unsure how to proceed without such instant discoveries then literally work your way through the chapters methodically, starting with Chapter 1 and moving on to the next chapter when you've developed a degree of familiarity and experiential skill. Almost certainly things will begin to join up as you proceed, so that by the time you get to the final chapter you will have developed a finesse and sensitivity that will enable you to have a deep and meaningful experience of your whole body that was previously unimaginable. Good luck.

Chapter 1

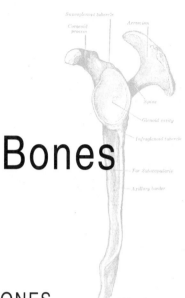

Bones

REFLECTIONS ON BONES – HUMOUR OR HORROR?

The skeleton is such a common image in our society. All those bones making up that familiar image of a full skeleton appearing mostly in scary movies, TV dramas, comedies and museums, conjuring up a whole mixture of feelings, but especially feelings of fear. I remember as a child watching the army of skeletons in *Jason and the Argonauts* and having nightmares about them. There was something inhuman and unnatural about them. For sure it's unnatural to have skeletons running around animated, but really, live humans aren't that much different. After all, half the body is the skeleton!

It's no wonder the skeleton is laughed at. It does look ridiculous on its own without all the other parts of the body to fill in the spaces. Despite its humorous affliction, the skeleton is often depicted as something dead and static. I wonder how all of this affects how we feel about our own living skeleton? Asking a few people what they thought about their skeleton, I got some fascinating responses: 'It feels weak', 'Lacking in support', 'Fragile', and also the opposite, 'It feels indestructible, hard and dense'.

The skeleton seems to exemplify the strangeness of the body and it can be difficult to equate 'ourselves' with it. My sense is that it commonly leads to feelings of fear and aversion, essentially towards our own death. Hence, understandably, for most people their sense of themselves is very different to the idea or image of a skeleton. There's a gap between how they may feel their own skeleton is inside of themselves and the visual image of it, so it becomes difficult to have a relationship with our skeletons.

Apart from this strangeness there's also the feeling that the hardest part of us can equally be quite vulnerable. It's certainly not indestructible, which is what we would like. We can worry about whether our bones are strong or hard enough to support us – and that's fair enough. The images that come to us can give us mixed messages about their strength. Maybe what I was really scared about in *Jason and the Argonauts* was how easily the skeleton soldiers were struck down.

WE ALL HAVE A SKELETON

Each one of us has our own. Just think about that. It sounds obvious, but it's not really something we ever think about or deeply consider. It's definitely part of who we are. In fact, it's about half of who we are, taken as a proportion of the whole body. The thing is that it's hidden within the body, out of sight – like many structures of our body we can't see and therefore have a poor relationship with. We manage to engage in quite a demanding relationship with the very outermost layer of our body: the skin and its contours. When you think about it, it's only when something terrible has happened that we are suddenly forced into a relationship with our bones. It's no wonder there's so much fear about the skeleton – when you see it there are often mortal consequences. The only other time we come closer to our skeleton is through illness or old age, when we often become skeletal. Bones start to show through our skin as the rest of the body's tissues waste away. We interpret this as a prelude to death; after all the harbinger of death, the Grim Reaper, is depicted as a skeleton.

How do we begin to sift through these difficult images and emotions in order to relate to the idea of healthy, living bones, of the *living* skeleton, not the skeleton of death or dying? In this society we hardly ever see death and maybe that's a strong part of our antipathy to bones. Our determination to keep death at bay creates a wealth of material for the unconscious to fantasize about: decaying bodies in graves, walking skeletons and horror movies eager to bring cemeteries to life. This chapter tries to encourage a healthy relationship to bones and in the process you may understandably meet some resistances in your own attempts; you may even feel and visualize images of death. It's a strange juxtaposition: the sight of our bones represents death, yet they are in fact the most alive and vital parts of ourselves, nurturing life. It's no wonder we can feel confused about our bodies. Try to hold on to the concept of the vibrant health that lies deep in your bones.

ARE BONES LIKE CONCRETE?

Bones are not rigid. You can test this by holding someone's forearm in two places (near the elbow and the wrist) and trying to bend it. You will notice that it bends. Bones do provide support for the softer parts of the body, but it's not as simple as that. The truth is that the body has a great natural strength throughout the whole of it, derived from the contribution of all tissues, like bones, muscles, blood vessels and nerves, but in particular from membranes. It's a mistake to consider our skeleton as a rigid structure that keeps us together and we wouldn't want our bones to be like concrete anyway. We'd be tough for sure but we'd lose so much of our natural flexibility and, in fact, it's our flexibility that allows for so much strength.

MIND AND BONES

Can the ideas we have about our bones shape how they are physically? Ideas can lead to feelings about ourselves that are often based on misperceptions and I'm interested in how these forces can affect us. Perhaps it can lead to a psychological mindset that affects how we relate to our body and that, in turn, shapes how we see the world. Most of us are so deeply influenced by these forces that they lead us to have a view of our body in an unconscious way. We receive ideas about bones as being concrete, fragile or scary. Can this affect the bones themselves? Do bones become dense and rigid because of our ideas of them? What does fear do to them? Can this lead to ill health and disease? Can this, in turn, lead us to suffer from mental density and rigidity? I believe it's important to consider these questions and really get to grips with some of the internal messaging we may be engaging with, albeit in an unconscious way. It would be healthier to know yourself than not. Can we have a relationship with our bones that leads us to health, longevity and revelation, rather than osteoporosis or arthritis?

FACTS ABOUT BONE

Bones are not steel girders. They are slightly bendy and full of movement from blood and nerve impulses. They are most definitely not static – if anything, they are highly active. Bones are formed from collagen fibre by adding calcium salts to create a blend of flexibility and toughness. The collagen provides a natural elasticity and the calcium a matrix of strong durable material. Throughout the bones there are spaces for small arteries and veins that supply the living cells situated in the bones with nutrients and oxygen. Most bones have a dense area immediately under the surface, and deeper into the interior the bone becomes less dense. These areas of the bone are called compact and spongy, respectively. Bones are white in the living body, not brown as in the dead version, because of collagen. Collagen is the most common substance in the body and is a protein that the body manufactures. It holds us together and gives us strength with 'bendiness' (more about this later). Cells in the bones constantly manufacture collagen and keep the bone renewed by making sure there's enough calcium deposited.

So you can see, bones need constant looking after. They are not like concrete that, once set, needs no attention. That's completely the wrong analogy. It takes a lot of energy for the cells to carry out their functions and for this they need a constant flow of food (i.e. blood). So there's a powerful flow of blood streaming through your bones all the time – gallons in a day. The other misconception people have is that we need calcium in large quantities otherwise our bones will become weak and disintegrate. Where did this obsession come from? The truth is that the body metabolizes calcium from everything we eat. Your body is a self-contained, efficient and regulating system.

SOME OBSERVATIONS ABOUT THE SKELETON

Spend a while looking at a picture of the skeleton. Look at it as if you have never seen it before. What do you observe? What are the things that strike you most? The first thing could simply be how strange and amazing it is. What else? Here are some of my observations. There are lots of bones made in different shapes. They are mostly arranged around a central axis called the spine. In some ways everything comes off the spine. The head is pivoted at the top of it, looking precarious. How does it balance on top of the slender cervical spine and why does it contain so much bone? (To protect the brain.) Look at the ribs. They all originate at the spine and form a cage. Why? Why has nature created so much bone here in such a formation? (To protect the heart, etc.) Then the rest is a pelvic and shoulder girdle, with limbs coming off each one, which are really quite similar to each other. Similar kinds of bones slightly modified for different uses. They are long bones, bigger in the legs.

The most important observation is that the skeleton is upright. This presents some huge problems that somehow we overcome all the time. Having a big brain helps to accomplish this and it's the reason why we have, proportionately, such a large head. Large parts of the brain provide smooth, precise controls on how we move. Probably a third of the brain is there for just this function!

GETTING TO KNOW YOUR BONES

The only way to really get to know your bones is to feel them. You can obviously feel them through your skin and muscles with your hands, but you can also feel them through your internal senses. You are actually doing this all the time – it's just that you're not aware of it. Your bones are being monitored for their position and health through nerve receptors that detect changes in motion and pressure. Let's bring our attention to these senses and create a greater awareness of your bones. A useful way of learning how to feel something is to feel it in comparison to something else. Below are some exercises for feeling bone in comparison to other tissues in the body, feeling the power of bones and feeling the different kinds of bones in your body.

Exercise: Feeling bone

Put your hands on your thighs. Let your attention move to your hands and thighs. Your hands are very sensitive and can receive lots of information about movement and tone. Can you get a sense of the skin? How taut it is and how it forms a container for the rest of the tissues in the thigh. Deepen your awareness to take in the muscle. Notice the difference in feeling. Muscle has a very different quality to it because it is formed quite differently. Let your awareness deepen even more until you get a sense of the bone right at the centre of the thigh. How does it feel? Can you get a sense of its quality? It is much denser and made up of different substances. Be open to feeling the whole bone. It's a long bone running from the hip to the knee. Let your awareness broaden out to include the whole bone. Stay with the sense of it for a while and see what comes to you.

Stay with your sensations for as long as possible. Don't dismiss your instinctive responses. Now, can you get a sense of movement within the bone? Can you sense deep within the bone? Into the marrow? The marrow is a powerful place in the body. It's where your blood and immune cells are made and where you store fat for energy. In oriental medicine it's a place where your energy is meant to be at its most powerful. Sit with that thought and stay with the sense of the marrow. Blood is constantly moving through the bone into the marrow so you might even get a strong sense of blood flow.

MORE ABOUT BONES

Bones come in lots of different shapes, sizes and densities. The bones found in the limbs and rib cage are called 'long bones' because they are long. Equally there are bones called 'short

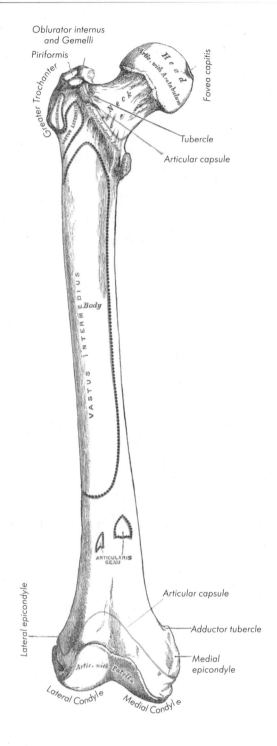

bones' for that very reason. Sometimes anatomists do name things in simple terms, but for the most part, it's a very complex and strange terminology. Short bones are mostly found in the hands and feet. Other bones are 'irregular shaped' which is mostly the uniquely bony spine. Then we come to the head, which is a totally unique and different structure to the rest of the body. Interestingly, bones in the rest of the body are covered by muscles, but the head is more like an exoskeleton. Most of the head is solid hard whereas the rest of the body is soft followed by hard underneath. The ribs are hard first, but not solid. It's good to understand these structures in simplistic terms as it allows us to get an immediate sense of their purpose.

The head comes in three parts: the face, which is a complex structure and therefore referred to as the 'facial complex', with 15 bones involved in it; the top of the head which has six bones and the base of the head which has four. It makes sense that the face is so complex because it's where a lot of movements take place – seeing, smelling, eating, breathing, talking. A mammoth task requiring a complex nerve supply. It's got specially created cranial nerves that control it – 12 pairs of them! That's a lot. They control all the movements and sensations that occur in the face with fine, delicate control of many of the unique muscles for expression. All of that takes up a lot of space in the brain. The bones in the face are amazing. Take a look at some of their shapes (see page 26).

It's interesting to think that this is what we're looking at most of the time. Bizarrely shaped bones that lie just beneath the skin and muscles of the face. The pointy one is called the vomer, which means plough, and it sticks directly forward from the centre of the face. Then there's the maxillae (two of them) that double-handedly make up most of the centre of the face, also creating the roof of the mouth and at the same time the floor of the nose and sinuses. They also form the sides of the

Bones of the face

nose, the lower part of the eye orbit and the upper teeth. That's a lot of things for a bone to do! So I vote them the most multitasking bones in the body! The other remarkable structures are the eye sockets (proper name orbit). Each orbit is made up of seven bones. That's an incredible amount of bones relating to each other to make a perfect circle. Incredibly, they do just

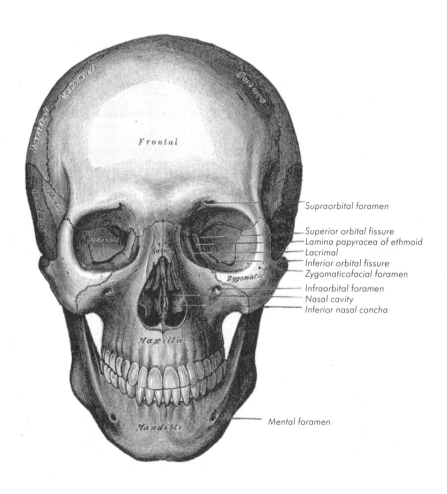

Supraorbital foramen

Superior orbital fissure
Lamina papyracea of ethmoid
Lacrimal
Inferior orbital fissure
Zygomaticofacial foramen

Infraorbital foramen
Nasal cavity
Inferior nasal concha

Mental foramen

that – the vast majority of the time. Sure, there's often a little variation in the size of our orbits, but mostly they grow to the same size.

Exercise: Feel what's in your face

The pad of your second finger is the most sensitive, so use it to explore the bony orbit around your eye. If you do it delicately you will feel the joins between the bones. These are unique joints called sutures. If you start from the corner of the eye next to the nose and work your way along the top of the eye orbit it should feel smooth. That's because there are no joints there. As you come down to the diagonal corner you should feel a bump or ridge as you move from the frontal bone to the cheekbone. Then, move your finger along the lower edge of the orbit and you should feel another bump as you move into the maxilla. Notice also how the bone density changes. It's really thick on the top and much thinner along the lower part of the orbit.

The rest of the head is next to the face and is called the neurocranium because it covers the brain – it's really that simple. It's made up of thin, flat plate-like domed bones starting off life as membranes, then ossifying (really good word for 'becoming bone') pre and post birth. It's useful to have soft membranous-like bones for being born. These bones are here to protect the brain and there's a trade-off between strength and mobility – if they were too thick and heavy you would not be able to hold your head up and move it around easily. To increase suppleness the muscles in the neck are kept to a minimum and this is important for survival. Thick bones like, for instance, the rhinoceros has are great for protection, but just look at the size of its neck muscles. Doesn't make for supple, flexible movements. It's wonderful to learn and observe the trade-offs our body nature makes. Standing upright means the head can weigh only so much. The sheer mechanics of supporting a heavy object at the top of the spine predetermine the size of the rest of the body. Thick cranium equals heavy head, equals bigger more powerful body to support it, means less mobility and suppleness. Such a big brain needs suppleness, which means that the body is less able to provide the brain with information about its environment. So there is protection offered with light bones on the roof of the brain and thicker heavier bones on the floor of the brain. Some of the thicker bones have air spaces in them (sinuses) to make it all a bit lighter (also for sound resonance so we can hear ourselves speak).

Exercise: Know your cranium

The best way to find the cranial bones is to find the suture lines first, as they are so large and prominent. The frontal bone is the biggest bone. It forms the top of the eyes and the front of the head – back beyond the hairline. You can find its joint by placing your thumb pads just in front of that funny, flappy bit at the front of your ear, and then turning your hands around so you bring your first fingertips together at the top of your head. This is where you would wear a tiara if you were a princess. Right underneath this line is the coronal suture. Feel it with your fingers by running them across that line. It can feel quite jagged and rough. As you come to the top of the head you will find the space where the fontanelle was when you were born. This is often very sensitive so don't press too strongly. Move your fingers directly back from this place along the sagittal suture. This is comb-like in shape and reaches into the back of the head where it forks into two suture lines moving down to the sides of the back of the head. There's one more major suture that runs around the top of the ears in a big curve and is called the squamous suture. This is much smoother and not so easy to feel.

When you've got a sense of the sutures you can start to have a sense of the bones. Put both of your palms on the top of your head. Move them forwards and backwards slightly, feeling the whole of the top of the head. Now move your hands down the sides, down to ear level, then down to the bottom of the ear. Similarly move your hands to the front of the head, up to the eyes and down the back of the head to the top of the neck. What do you notice? It's clear that the bones on the top of the head are much thinner than the bones at the base of the head. It feels softer on top and harder below. Notice how your body responds to your enquiring hands. Is there a difference in sensitivity or quality in the various areas?

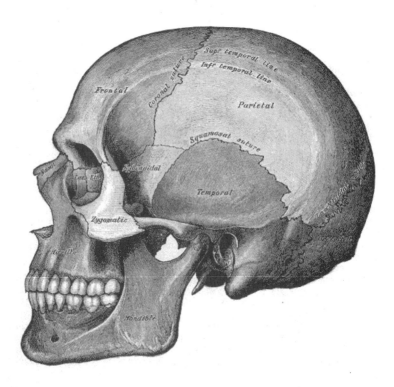

THE ELEMENTS IN YOUR BONES

Calcium makes up most of your bones and is also the sixth most abundant element in the earth's crust. Of all the structures in your body, bones contain the most non-organic material making bone a unique tissue in the body. If you listen to your bones you can feel the connection to the earth.

When you look at it more closely, deposits of various calcium salt crystals make up about two-thirds of the weight of bone, the other third coming from collagen fibres (made from protein – more about them later), with only 2 per cent of bone consisting of living cells. This phenomenon of living tissue co-existing with non-organic substances running throughout the body makes for a very curious relationship. Actually most of the body is formed of extracellular substances and not living tissue. Or to put it another way, cells only constitute part of the body, and the rest is made up of non-cellular substances. The big question, therefore, is how alive is the body after all? Is it just cells that are alive that represent consciousness or are substances such as collagen protein and calcium salts conscious and alive in a special way, because they are in the body? If these were outside the body they would be considered dead bone, without the blood, the marrow or the bone cells. The general evidence is that cells control non-cellular substances and that these substances are functional, but not intelligent, but maybe that's not quite the whole truth. The exercises above reveal a strong sense of presence in bones, certainly a strong sense that they belong to you and are not dead substance. Don't forget when you feel bones that just 2 per cent of the bone is cells and the rest is non-cellular. Something to reflect upon.

So you can see that the body is made up of quite a few elements like calcium that exist in combination with other elements. Some of them are surprising. For instance, hydrogen is the most abundant element in the body (62%), followed by oxygen (26%), then carbon (10%) and nitrogen (1.5%). So are we carbon-based units after all? Seems to me more like hydrogen-based. What's interesting is that three of the most abundant elements are gases. Oxygen and nitrogen are the major constituents of air, and hydrogen is mostly what the sun is made of. The rest of the elements all come from the ground. Apart from carbon, which is easily the most abundant of these, these are minerals and metals from the ground and only make up 1 per cent of the body. So we are made mostly of sun and air with small parts of the earth. Calcium, even though it's throughout our bones, only makes up 0.2 per cent of the body and iron just 0.0005 per cent, so let's not get too carried away about taking in calcium and iron when what we really need is oxygen, carbon and hydrogen!

However, with all that in mind (and it's pretty mind-blowing), since your bones contain the greatest quantity (remember two-thirds of the weight of bone) of elements and non-organic material from the earth, it makes them a very good vehicle to feel the connection to the earth. In this way, by connecting to your bones you're immediately connecting to the stuff that made the planet in the first place and this facilitates a strong resonance. So, the next time you feel 'un-grounded', try thinking about your bones and here's an exercise to try and help you to do just that.

Exercise: Feeling the earth through your bones

Now that you have more of a sense of the elemental connectivity of the earth through your bones, let's try connecting to the earth through your body by bringing all of your bones into contact with it. Find a bit of earth to lie on. It could be in your garden or a park. Lie on your back, let your bones sink into the earth. Lie still and concentrate on the weight of your bones dropping into the earth and you will start to notice how earthy you really are. Let your bones resonate with the earth below you. Notice how you feel. If you stay with this longer you will feel intrinsically part of it, as if you are dissolving into the ground. Consider the calcium in your bones merging with the ground below you and observe what happens.

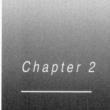

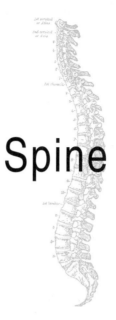

Chapter 2

Spine

The spine is the core of the body's structure and it's the first aspect of you to be formed in the womb. The next page shows an image of the spine. Pretend you haven't seen it before and stare at it for a while with an open mind. What are you struck by? Make a list of some simple observations that grab your curiosity.

Here's what I see. First, it's curved, smooth at the front and knobbly at the back. It tapers to the top. It's thicker at the bottom, and ends in one large triangular bone. The overall sense is of something prehistoric. The really big thing is that it's within my body.

WHY IS IT CURVED?

When you were forming yourself, at around the third week of your life, you curled up along your whole length and went from being flat and straight to being curved (that familiar foetal position). Later, after birth, at around six months old, you began to look up from the floor, preparing to crawl. The first

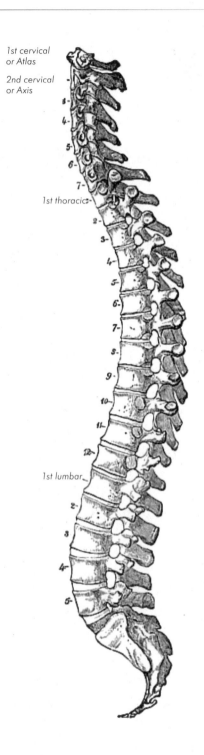

1st cervical
or Atlas

2nd cervical
or Axis

1st thoracic

1st lumbar

The spine

event created the curve of the spine in the upper back and the curve of the spine in the pelvis, which have remained curved the same way since. The curves in your neck and lower back were created when you looked up and pushed your hands into the floor. This gives the spine the ability to curve in both directions, front and back. It also gives it some of the qualities of a spring, though it does reach an optimum curviness. If the spine is too flat and poker-like, it is difficult to move and balance weight. Too curvy, and it can equally create strain, especially at the bottom of the spine where there is more weight to bear. A healthy spine is spring loaded. It cushions the impact of sudden or strenuous movement. All vertebrates have this ability, but for man it's more critical because we stand upright.

Let's look at the mechanics of the spine. There's an awesome balancing act that happens between the head and the top of the spine. Really take a moment to appreciate this. Delicate balancing mechanisms create fine control around the top of the spine, as well as along the whole length of the spine, and your entire posture shifts and adjusts to allow the head to remain within this balance tolerance. A large portion of the brain and many tiny muscles in the neck and top of the spine are actively engaged in this process.

Just a little further down are the ribs hanging off the spine. They all connect directly with it. At a certain stage of our embryological development, our ribs originated at the spine and then grew out to the sides and forward. It's quite an impressive structure and, in fact, all that weight would be easier to carry if we were still on all four limbs. Hence, walking upright presents a much more demanding challenge which our brains constantly compensate for by keeping a tight control of how we walk and hold ourselves through a multitude of nerve impulses and muscles.

WHY IS THE SPINE KNOBBLY AND SMOOTH?

The spine is smooth at the front and knobbly at the back. The knobbly bits are for our protection and provide an excellent place for muscles to attach. There's an astonishing number of muscles that attach here – in fact, there are more muscles in the spine than the rest of the body put together. There's a good reason for this as there are more joints in the spine than anywhere else in the body, which endows the spine with great mobility. This mobility is facilitated by all these muscles and an efficient nerve supply to inform them. Those knobbly bits pointing straight back are a bit like a stegosaurus, and looking at the spine you kind of feel like there's something ancient to it. If you run your fingers down someone's spine you can feel all those pointy tips, right from the top to the bottom, ending at the coccyx. There are typically 26. You can find knobbly bits that point out to the sides as well, but they are much more difficult to feel – the easiest place to feel them is in the neck, if you feel deeply into the sides of the neck.

The smooth part is at the front of the spine, deep in the centre-back of the chest and abdominal cavities. It's made up of blocks of solid bone called vertebrae. We tend to think of the spine as being at the back of the body, but that's just the tips of the spine. The spine is actually very much part of the front of the body too. You'll find many internal muscles and structures that attach to it within the chest and abdomen, so the spine is an integral part of both the front and the back of the body. It's useful to contemplate this because, in a sense, the spine is looking internally at the front yet, at the back, it's looking out to the world. That's quite a view!

TENSEGRITY

You get a sense of how the spine is held not only by the bony spinal column, but also by the contribution of many different muscles, ligaments and membranes, all acting together to give the core of the body its qualities. This inter-relationship between all these different tissues is what we refer to as tension integrity or 'tensegrity'. Tension integrity is not only about the quality of our joints (as many people think), but also about having the right muscle tone to be supple (i.e. to have fluid and elastic qualities). For many of us we lose these 'fluid-like' qualities and become dehydrated and fixed. Less mobile. As you get older you can avoid this through a combination of correct diet, exercise, rest, posture and state of mind. The more fluid and elastic you are the more likely you are to be vital and creative. Often, how the body is, so the mind follows. What is a vital and creative, fluid and elastic mind like? The answer is, a mind that can truly think. Thinking requires a willingness to look at all perspectives, a certain amount of flexibility in all circumstances. Our imagination helps us to achieve this. If there's fixity in your body, your mind will be under a lot of pressure to follow suit. See if you can observe this in your daily life. Linear and absolutist ways of thinking often miss the whole complexity of the inter-relatedness of all things, and thereby produce systems that imitate this way of thinking. Systems that can be rigid and limiting as opposed to systems that can be supple or have an integrity towards a multiplicity of relationships. If we come back to the image of a healthy spine, we could say that how the healthy spine works, with all its intricate relationships, could offer a blueprint for business, society, relationships and the environment.

Exercise: Finding your spine 1

Imagine your attention/awareness is like fluid. Let it flow down from your head, along the length of your spine, right into the bottom of the spine in the pelvis. Sensations of your spine will come to you. Try to feel the knobbly bits, the curves, bones and the spine as a unit. That's really the important thing – bringing your awareness to the whole spine. It's composed of many separate parts, but the overall nature of the spine is that it's one unit of function. We can forget this and get lost in the bits and pieces of it. Find your whole spine again and you will find your relationship to the whole of you. This is the way to 'holistic relationship'. A whole relationship with yourself, people, nature and the universe at large. How important is this? Spend some time making this relationship with your spine and observe what happens in your life. Finding your spine is transformative.

WHY IS YOUR SPINE THE MOST AMAZING THING IN THE UNIVERSE?

You could argue that the brain is far more impressive than the spine, but, when you think about it, the brain just sits in a bony ball doing its neural thing, waiting for the world to come to it. In a way, the spine does that too, but through movement it also gets out into the world. In many ways the spine is also a brain – it's even got white and grey matter – and yet it moves, all the time, like a snake. What is just so totally awesome is that something as delicate as your nervous system is able to be held within the largest moving part of the body! It's the communication highway of the body and, simultaneously, it's the anchor for all the body's structures. A wonderful balance is created between mechanical, hydraulic and electro-chemical actions. That, in itself, is totally awe inspiring, but it doesn't end there. Most of the body's movements take place from the spine, directly or indirectly. It also contains the central nervous system, special fluids, half the bones and most of the joints in the body, has a complex arrangement of muscles and all the organs cluster around it. QED It's amazing!

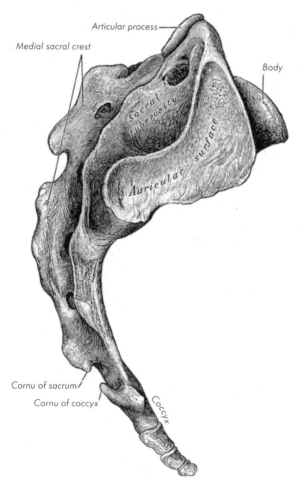

The sacrum

Exercise: Finding your spine 2

Sitting, allow your awareness to come into your spine. Notice how your spine feels. Notice how your head sits on top of your spine. Perhaps you are aware of your head rotating or bending to one side. See what happens if you move your head into a different position in relationship to the spine in the neck.

Do the same thing for your shoulders. Take your time. Orienting your shoulders in different ways will change how the spine in your chest aligns itself. See if you can feel these relationships.

Look/feel for a better sense of your centre line – the relationship from the head through the spine into the pelvis. Feeling this centre line results in a better distribution of the weight of the head and body down the spine into the sacrum.

Now, standing up, slowly adjust the angle of your pelvis side to side and rotate the pelvis front to back. Notice if your body weight is conveyed/transmitted more easily through the sacro-iliac joints into the major weight-bearing joints of the legs.

Adjust your leg stance. Notice if your weight is supported more through one leg than the other. Again, try to come into a more powerful sense of your centre line/centre of gravity through the whole spinal axis of the body, down through the legs into the feet.

Just sit for a while after this. Let your mind relax and notice how you feel generally, what state of mind and emotions you are in, and also how you feel in relation to the space around you.

SPINE AS A SPRING

Springs have coiled energy in them and this creates the potential for springiness. If you bring an image of a spring to your mind, how does it make you feel? You know if you press the end of the spring it will either push back at you with strength or it will try to curve away. This is how the healthy spine should feel to you, like it has an internal energy that can resist gravity. Thinking about your spine in this way really changes your relationship to it. Keeping your spine in motion will really help to keep its bounce. You can imagine that lack of motion might cause some of the coils to get stuck together and the spine's movement as a whole would become sticky, reducing its overall springiness. So, keep your spine alive by bouncing!

Exercise: Learning to bounce

Standing with your feet hip-width apart, let your body relax. Stand like this for a while and try to feel your spine. What does it feel like? Does it feel evenly balanced throughout its length? Does it feel springy? Or does it feel stiff or painful? Maybe it doesn't feel like anything, particularly. That's fine. In any case, slowly allow your spine to begin to bounce. To do this, you need to move up and down along the length of your body. Initially, most of the movement comes from the joints in the legs bending and flexing, but as you proceed you will notice that your spine starts to move like a concertina along its length. Let your shoulders relax. This will allow the spine in your neck to move more freely. Let your shoulder blades drop and soften the area between them. This should allow your upper spine in the chest to move more freely. Let your belly muscles relax. This will allow your lower spine and pelvis to move more freely. Keep going. Don't do it too roughly. Try to be gentle and subtle with the bouncing and you will find that after ten minutes the spine starts to come alive and it can feel like the bounce is coming from within it. Try holding the image of a springy coil in your mind's eye if it helps you. The more often you practise this exercise, the springier your spine will become and the more youthful you will feel. You can notice how children and animals have this natural spring in them and you'll be amazed when you regain this through practice.

SPINE AS YOUR HISTORY – CHANGING HISTORY

More than any other structure in your body, it's your spine that defines who you are, even more than your face or personality. I believe that on a deep unconscious level most people know this, and often judgements and assessments are made of others by the position of their posture. Your spine holds your history and reveals how you have lived your life. That's why body therapists such as osteopaths, chiropractors and physiotherapists inspect it. It shows health and trauma. Simplistically, suppleness reveals health, whereas lack of movement, anywhere along its length, informs us that the spine has been compromised in that segment in some way. The most common examples are the lower spine becoming compressed, affecting digestion, or the spine at the bottom of the ribs becoming stiff and immobile, affecting breathing, or the top of the spine becoming sore and tense, affecting how we think. These symptoms can arise from injuries or build up over a period of time through bad posture, or they can arise from reactions to emotional stress, or just simply feeling overtaxed or overburdened by life – a part of your spine will physically respond to the stress by tightening up. Whole layers of difficult experiences can be logged along the length of the spine and slowly the spine loses its natural qualities. I'm certain we all have experience of this. So, change your spine and you change your history. Bring your spine together as a unit and you will bring yourself out of your fragmented history and into the present. It's important to recognize that when the spine becomes taxed and overburdened, it loses its integrity to be whole, and instead it becomes a series of isolated vertebrae relating only to themselves or just to their immediate neighbours. As a result, you become fragmented in your person and in your life. This is unhealthy and is a low energy state. It's almost as if the spine has become sunken under the weight of personal history. You can roll back time by bringing your spine back into wholeness through the use of awareness and movement.

THE SPINE AND THE UNIVERSE

Looking at an image of the spine, it's obvious to see that it mimics the form of a wave with undulating crests and troughs. The universe communicates in different frequencies of waves, whether from light, sound, energy, water or matter. I believe we have been made in this likeness to connect and communicate with the universal laws of nature. If you consider our core to be a wave, it's almost as if it is designed to be a receptacle to specifically receive similar wave-like signals from our environment. Since we receive information from nature, people and the environment on a continual basis, surely it makes sense that this very structure of communication, the spine, would therefore absorb and reflect the same wave-like form that the universe adopts.

We often refer to our instinctive responses as 'coming from the gut', but we feel things in our spine as well, as vibrations. In fact, one could argue that our gut responds to an impulse from our spine. The best way to consider this would be to remember how integrated and connected all these structures are, so, in reality, your gut is not separate from your spine. Hence, it would be fair to conclude that the suppler, bouncier and healthier your spine is, the more instinctually wise you would become. The more receptive you are, the more informed your decisions can be. That way, you would make clearer choices about your relationships and be able to determine a way of life that is compatible for you.

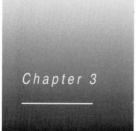

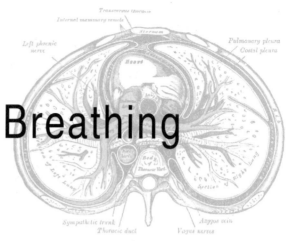

Chapter 3

Breathing

The mysterious, crazy, wonderful thing about life is the way we take so many things for granted. For example, the way we live on a spinning globe that moves around a huge fiery ball, or how we walk, think or breathe. Breathing in particular. For many of us, breathing is just this thing that happens in the background, and yet the two biggest movements in the body are the heart beating and breathing. Nature kindly filters these movements out from our normal consciousness, as otherwise we would be overwhelmed and unable to think, make decisions or function as an intelligent sentient being. The crazy bit is that we can develop a total lack of awareness of either of these vital movements and become oblivious to the state of our body, which has great consequences for our health. Our body becomes overwhelmed and dysfunctional, because we are not paying enough attention to the signals it's sending us. By bringing your attention to your breath, you might notice that it's not full enough or deep enough. This is an important signal as it indicates that you are therefore not delivering sufficient oxygen to your cells. This results in a loss of energy and efficiency throughout your whole system (not to mention your body needing to break itself down to create energy for its basic functions).

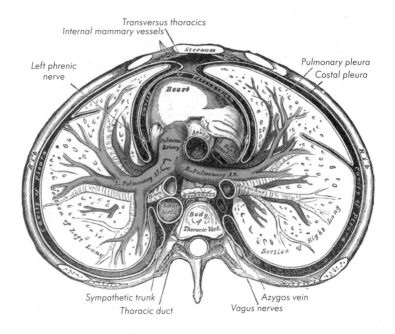

The pulminary circuit

How can we lose connection to such a vital force as our breathing? Why does this happen? I've noticed a few reasons over the years, the most common being:

- stress

- depression

- unexpressed emotions

- poor posture

- learnt habits

- lack of body awareness.

The problem is that we get so used to overriding the body's signals that we no longer even notice them. Most people, when asked how their breathing is, look slightly bewildered and then shrug their shoulders and answer 'fine' or 'ok', as if it's obvious or inconsequential. It's only when you begin to question them in more detail about their breathing that you start to hear more informed answers, like 'it's a bit shallow sometimes' or 'I notice I hold my breath'. It can take many sessions of these questions along with breathing awareness exercises to get all the detail. When you have this detail you are back in relationship with your body's communication about how it is – it's the body's sensory nervous system that's telling you this. You've stopped overriding and can now feel/sense how you breathe. You will come to know just how huge a thing it is in your life – in your body, mind and emotions. Your breathing is at the very centre of your life, and the mechanism enabling this life-giving act is rarely understood or fully appreciated. People tend to think of breathing as an operation that occurs simply in the lungs, but it's the diaphragm, one of the biggest structures in your body, that controls your every breath.

THE DIAPHRAGM

The diaphragm is so big it divides our torso into two halves, literally forming two cavities. It's a big flat muscle used for breathing and is shaped like a bell. Its highest point on the centre line of the body is at the level of the bottom of the breast-plate. Place your fingers on your breast-plate (or sternum) and feel down its length. When you come to the bottom you will notice a sticky-out bony bit that can feel blunt or pointed. That's your ziphoid process, and just behind it is where the diaphragm attaches to the sternum. From there it runs along the inside of the ribs, angling down towards the back of the body, doming into the spine at the level of the last ribs. You can feel your ribs using your thumbs, pressing along them at the back until you come to the last rib. If you follow it out to the sides of the body, you will feel it is quite short and has a pointy

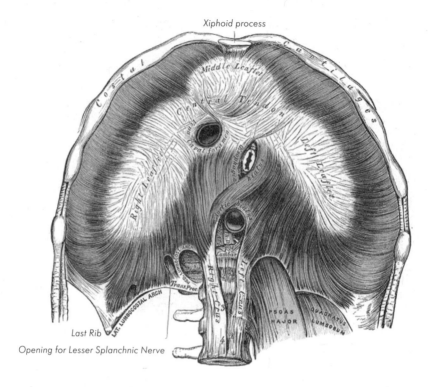

Xiphoid process

Last Rib

Opening for Lesser Splanchnic Nerve

The diaphragm

tip that can be tender. This is a floating rib. Put one hand at the ziphoid process (bottom of breast-plate) and the other hand on the last rib and you will notice that the two hands are about six inches apart. That's how much the diaphragm domes! The diaphragm also has strands of muscle moving from its centre-back area, reaching down along the spine, to the level of your navel and slightly below. When you see pictures of these strands they look like the roots of the diaphragm. So that means the diaphragm connects from the breast-plate of the chest to the spine at navel level. That's an extraordinary distance!

On the upper surface of the diaphragm sits the heart and the bottom of both lungs. On its underside, the liver, stomach and spleen are in intimate contact with it, and at the back the kidneys. The diaphragm is also intimately related to the spine and the rib cage.

THE HEALTHY DIAPHRAGM

The diaphragm flattens to create a vacuum in the lungs for inhalation. It domes on exhalation. If this movement is reduced through tension or strain then breathing will be reduced along with mobility of organs as well as the spine. The diaphragm is responsible for 75 per cent of breathing (the rest is rib breathing from intercostal muscles). Tension can therefore greatly reduce the intake of air and expulsion of carbon dioxide. Shallow breathing is a product of this. When the diaphragm moves healthily, it massages all the internal organs and allows passage of blood, lymph, food and nervous impulses through it. It also allows the spine to be more mobile and flexible. Typically, when the diaphragm flexes, it will widen side to side and move down, increasing the pressure in the abdominal cavity. This results in a massaging of the abdominal organs, helping to move fluids and facilitate many physiological processes; in particular, helping blood to return to the heart from the lower body. It is for this reason that the diaphragm is often described as the second heart.

Exercise: Exploring your diaphragm

Place your hands on the front of your chest. Follow your breath through your nose into your chest. Notice how your rib cage moves. How much does it move? It should rise and widen on the in-breath. You may notice places within it that are resistant to movement. Shoulders should rise and fall in a relaxed manner. Try and feel your ribs moving. Do they all move?

Then move your hands down to the bottom of the sternum – to the level of the top of the diaphragm. See if you can have an internal sense of the diaphragm doming and flattening – it's a natural movement. How much movement does it make? It's so big you can't miss it.

Focus on your breathing and notice if the diaphragm softens and if that changes your breathing, your spine, sense of your body or your state of mind. Encourage your diaphragm to soften by consciously letting go of it and relaxing as you breathe. Just bringing your hands to this part of the body is often enough to relax the muscles and connective tissues of the diaphragm, along with the organs on either side of it.

As you start to get more attuned to the movements of the diaphragm and your breathing, notice how much pressure there is in your abdomen on the in-breath. When you are breathing well you can feel it in your pelvic floor! It feels like the abdomen is inflating.

Bring your other hand to the back of the diaphragm (behind the navel) and notice how much your lower spine moves in response to your breathing. Keep listening with your hands and you will notice the curves of the spine shift and change in response to your in- and out-breaths. If your breathing is healthy, your whole spine joins in and all the curves deepen with the in-breath. Move your hand from the lower back area and place it on the back of your neck. Notice how your neck responds to the movements of your diaphragm. There are muscles in your neck that assist with raising your rib cage on the in-breath and you might feel muscles tensing under your hand. The curvature of the spine here also deepens on the in-breath.

LIFE CHANGING CONCLUSIONS

Now that you have listened to your diaphragm and learnt about your spine in the previous chapter, you can perhaps appreciate the connection between how you breathe and how your posture is. That's such an important relationship to understand. *Your breath and your posture are totally connected.* Poor breathing, poor posture. Healthy breathing, balanced posture. Just knowing that could change your life. Balanced posture and healthy breath are all you need in life to have energy, efficiency and confidence.

When you breathe well, you allow your diaphragm to massage your organs. This helps your organs function better. Your gut is helped with moving food through it, from the stomach to the intestines. You can feel your stomach being squeezed down on the in-breath (which it is!). Try tuning into this when you breathe. The diaphragm encourages a downwards movement that helps move digested food through the small intestine and works together with the natural movements of peristalsis (muscular action of the gut that moves food along its length). You can imagine that if your breathing is poor then your digestion could also be poor. That's also such an important link to make in your life. The two tend to go together. Good breathing, good digestion. Good digestion, good energy. Good energy, happy life. Happy means good breathing. Happy means you eat healthily and digest well.

When you breathe well, blood returning from the lower part of your body (i.e. below the heart, which is most of your body) is powerfully helped by your diaphragm's movements. The diaphragm, therefore, also acts as a pump for helping blood move through the main highway of blood returning to the heart – the inferior vena cava. This big vessel passes through the diaphragm, slightly on the right side, and all the veins of the legs and abdomen feed into it. It's like a slow river running up through the centre of you. Because it's so far from the heart's pumping action the movement relies on valves in the veins to stop backflow, along with muscular activity, hence the more activity you have the better. Sedentary lifestyle doesn't help. With every breath you take, the diaphragm (the biggest muscle in the body) squeezes blood through the vena cava. You can now understand why the diaphragm acts as the heart for the venal blood system.

Poor breathing can hinder blood returning to the heart, which in turn can lead to congestion in blood capillaries, water retention in the lower body, poor exchange processes across cell membranes and decreased metabolism. All of this reduces your energy and efficiency and you can start to feel heavy and lethargic. Not great.

Let's now also take a look at how upper body tension in the neck and shoulders can play havoc with your breathing. The muscles of your shoulders and neck must be open to move when your rib cage rises and widens. Your neck must be open to changing its curve. If your neck is stiff and tight your head will not be able to move in response to your breath. It becomes static and out of relationship with your body. The nerve that innervates the diaphragm exits the spinal cord in the neck and travels down the neck over the heart into the diaphragm. It's called the phrenic nerve. Here's a handy mnemonic to remember that 'C3, C4, C5 (cervical vertebrae 3, 4, 5) – keeps the diaphragm alive'. Of course, this can easily be affected by neck tension and rigidity.

JUST A REMINDER

It's very difficult to be perfectly in balance around your breathing. We all live lives that can produce difficult and challenging times and this will be reflected in your body, and particularly in your breathing. Stress can lead us all to shallow breathe at times and, through tension, we can place our bodies under varying degrees of pressure. The aim of this chapter is to encourage and empower you to bring awareness to your breathing and to understand the factors that influence your breathing. Your breathing will improve as a result of doing these exercises and should you be in a state of stress, they will help you to quickly come back to an optimal state. However, doing these exercises won't necessarily lead to perfect breathing – that depends on the bigger picture of what's going on in your life.

FURTHER EXPLORATIONS OF YOUR DIAPHRAGM

When you've made some discoveries using the above exercises and guidelines you might want to try the following exercises to deepen your understanding.

Exercise: More on posture

Standing up, bring your awareness to your feet and notice if there is any shift in weight across or along your feet as you breathe in and out. Can you tell what happens to the weight in your feet as you breathe? There is clearly a shift in weight as you breathe. Increased abdominal pressure and curving of the spine produces a movement of your centre of gravity forward from your navel. This produces a natural movement into the balls of the feet on the in-breath and into the heels on the out-breath. If this is not happening then check out what's going on in your pelvis and legs. Maybe there are places of tension that are preventing this. The pelvic floor and knees are common places to hold tension, but it's often quite individual. Ask yourself, ask your body, why this tension is being held.

If you can feel this movement at the feet then notice how each foot responds. Is there any difference? What does this tell you?

Similarly, feel what your head does as you breathe. Does it move? Which way and how? Healthy heads move subtly in response to the diaphragm.

These exercises can lead to heightened body awareness and a natural change in posture, so doing them as often as possible would be well worth your while.

Exercise: More on your organs

The diaphragm not only massages the gut, but the liver and the kidneys. Let's check this out by following how these organs respond to the breath.

Bring both your hands to your chest and find the bottom of your sternum and then the solar plexus – the soft area just below. Place your left hand on your solar plexus and your right hand along the edge of the rib cage on the right. Let the fingertips of the hands touch, so that the wrist of your right hand is facing out, towards the side of the ribs. Underneath both your hands and under the ribs is your liver. Big, eh? It is, in fact, the biggest single structure in the body. Now see if you can get a sense of it. Do this by following the movement of your diaphragm. Notice how the liver gets displaced downwards on the in-breath. If you are breathing well it should move a few inches. This is a critical movement for the liver's function. The liver is attached to the diaphragm by ligaments that bind it structurally to the diaphragm. So, where the diaphragm goes the liver follows.

Now slide your hand to the bottom of the rib cage at the back of your body. Find the floating ribs and know that each kidney is pretty much half covered by these ribs. The rest of the kidney is below the last rib. The diaphragm curves down as it moves towards the back of the body and the kidneys end up being close to it. It's strange to think that the kidneys are so near to the breathing apparatus. Follow your breath and notice how the kidneys respond. Are they moved by it? Keep the palm of each hand over a kidney. You can't miss them as they are so hot with blood. The movement of the diaphragm helps the kidneys in their function of removing waste from the blood.

THE DIAPHRAGM IN CONTEXT

Whole body bellowing

It helps to imagine that right at the centre of your body is a bellows, moving all day and all night. Never stopping till you die. It fans the digestive fire, creates heat in the body, helps the heart in transporting blood and helps the nervous system move into states of rest or activity. When we are stressed our breathing can, more than any other factor in the body, bring our internal state back to a steady state. Just like a bellows, the diaphragm can fan the fire in an easy paced way that lets the body's physiology run smoothly, or it can fan too strongly so that the body's system becomes too activated and energized. If this is too strong, the breathing can become erratic and lead to overactivation of the nervous system, and you can get symptoms like panic breathing, where the nervous system is out of control. Conversely, if there's poor breathing and the internal fire is not fanned, there is not enough energy for many necessary functions. This leads to low energy states.

Emotional and mental processing

When the diaphragm moves healthily it can help emotions process and resolve, creating a way for the body's emotions to balance. The rhythm of the diaphragm helps steady your emotional flux. Thought processes become smooth and the mind calm. This is a natural process. Look at babies – they can quickly change their emotional state if they are breathing healthily. When there is constriction in your breathing, emotions can become held in the body and difficult to express and your thinking becomes cloudy and chaotic.

Healthy relationships

Have you ever considered what the effects might be in our relationships if we allowed ourselves to breathe fully and let our diaphragm move freely? Might they begin to flourish? Restricted breathing means we aren't open or inviting and if we are too caught up inside ourselves, we don't move naturally outwards towards others. We become fearful and held in. You need to feel safe and at ease to move outwards into relationships. Only then can you effectively attach to others in a balanced way. So you could say, as your diaphragm is, so are your relationships to others, and, in a broader context, to the world, or life.

Diaphragmatic consciousness

If you think about it, when you establish a smooth, full movement of the diaphragm, your consciousness resonates with the diaphragm. Smooth, rhythmic, deep and powerful, yet hidden and understated, contained and internal. How would life be if we could approach the world in this way? A new level of awareness would start to manifest in your daily life that would allow you to be creative and remain in a state of dynamic interaction with your environment, relationships and internal needs. The diaphragm offers us the ultimate lesson in dynamic exchange, so keep listening.

Nature and the diaphragm

How can we let our breath resonate more with nature? I believe that as you deepen your connection to your breathing and diaphragm, you start to resonate with the natural forces of the environment. I'm often struck by how people who live rustic lives seem to be part of their surroundings. They exist within the natural rhythms of their environment and are healthier for it. There's a cohesion between their pace of life and the forces of nature around them. After all, is this not what city dwellers return to parks, forests and the countryside for – a boost of nature's vital energy? And the first place we notice this shift in our state of being is through our breath. Quite naturally, our breath settles. If we were able to connect to our breath in a deep and conscious way, I believe we would have immediate access to the deeper rhythms of life and this would influence our decisions, making them more consistent with the natural order of things.

Exercise: The sea and your diaphragm

For me, the diaphragm is like a tide machine moving the body in wave-like motion. Try testing this. Sit by the sea, or think of the sea, and let your diaphragm relax. Let a free connection take place and notice how your breath follows. Stay with this for a while and see if you can make a deeper connection to slower, deeper tide-like movements.

THE ORGANS OF BREATH

Now that we've understood the mechanism of the diaphragm, let's begin to see how our lungs are moved by it. The lungs are like trees turned inside out. The wind (our breath) doesn't move around the leaves and branches; it moves through the insides of them. The wind is the air we breathe in, the trunk is the trachea, the branches are the bronchi and the leaves are the alveoli. The trachea and bronchi are toughened with rings of strong cartilage that prevent them from collapsing, but the alveoli are very delicate. These are the structures we truly breathe through. They are shaped like a bunch of grapes at the end of the bronchial branches. Each grape is like a leaf. It's just one cell thick so that molecules can pass through it. On one side is air, on the other side is blood.

Exercise: Exploring your lungs

Sitting comfortably, bring your awareness to your nose (or mouth if you can't breathe through your nose) and feel the sensations the movement of air makes along both nostrils. Follow these sensations into the back of the nose. Here, there is a space where air from both nostrils meets, deep in the head, and moves down to the start of the trachea in the throat. Notice the change in sensations between the nostrils, the nasal cavity and the trachea. They all feel quite different – especially the trachea. You will be able to feel the movement of air divide as the trachea divides in two and starts to flow through the branches in both lungs. Feel how far down they go in the lungs. Let your awareness include the whole sensation from nose to alveoli. Notice how powerful a place the alveoli are. This is the interface between the external world and our internal environment. This is where we exchange gases – oxygen and carbon dioxide. At this interface there is a surface tension. Can you feel this in your lungs?

THE INTRICACIES OF THE RIB CAGE

The rib cage is literally a 'cage of ribs'. It's easy to forget this because we're so familiar with the term 'rib cage'. There are 24 curved bones of different sizes held together by tough cartilage at the front and by joints at the back of the body along the spine. As we breathe, the rib cage has to move with our breath via the joints along the spine. Take a few moments to appreciate this. The rib cage actually moves from the spine as we breathe and there are many muscles involved in order to do this. As you breathe in, the rib cage rises up and widens. Muscles in the shoulders and neck help the rising movement by tensing. Muscles between the ribs (the intercostals – meaning literally 'between the ribs') are mostly responsible for the widening and contracting of the ribs.

Exercise: Exploring your rib cage

Spend some time following the movements of your rib cage. Just notice the change in shape the rib cage makes through a full breath. It feels like the body is growing longer and wider on the in-breath. If you keep listening to the in-breath you might be able to feel the tensing of muscles in the neck, at the front of the chest and between the shoulder blades. These all work together to raise the rib cage. The widening is a movement that takes place from the joints in the spine. See if that's something you can recognize. It's as if you are opening out from your spine. Finally, move your awareness to the spaces between the ribs. These are the intercostal muscles. There are a few layers of muscles here that are responsible for the rising and descending of the rib cage. You might be able to feel the different sets of muscles tense on the in-breath and out-breath.

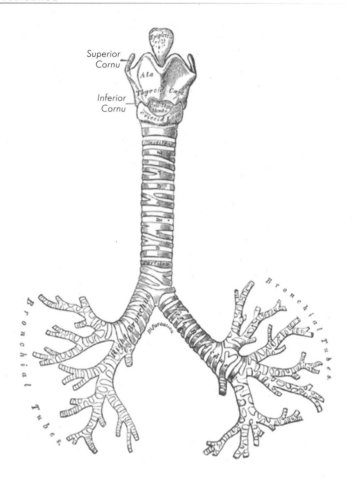

Superior Cornu

Inferior Cornu

The trachea (windpipe)

As you have probably gathered, breathing is a really big thing in our lives and hopefully this chapter has highlighted just exactly what is involved in the single act of taking oxygen in, transforming it and breathing carbon dioxide out. So many of our vital systems rely on the qualitative function of this process. It relates to and impacts on so many other organs and structures in the body that having a full understanding of this would only serve to help you appreciate the complexity and beauty of this mechanism, and never to take it for granted again.

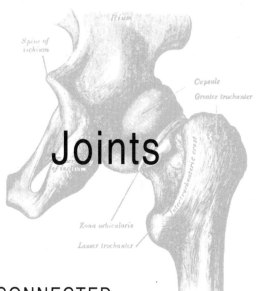

Chapter 4

Joints

KEEPING YOU CONNECTED

One way to look at the body is to see it divided into a myriad of small units all connected to each other, and the places where they meet would be our joints. Since our joints connect the whole body up, they are vital to the body staying in communication with itself and remaining whole.

A closer look at joints:

- A joint is a meeting place of bones, muscles, blood vessels and nerves.

- For every bone there are generally two joints.

- There are 206 bones in the body and 360 joints. So, you could say most of our body is to do with joints and how well we join ourselves up.

Joints are pretty much created in one of two ways, although most are of the first type:

Synovial joint: Between the bones there's a bag of egg-white fluid contained within a strong fibrous membrane. There's also a coating across the ends of the bones and ligaments that straddle the joint holding the bones together.

Fibrous joint: This refers to the disc joints we looked at in the chapter on the spine. More about these later.

Joints are massively important to our health and quality of life (secretly this is the most important chapter in the book). In many ways, you could assess your overall health by checking the mobility of your joints. If you can keep flexible and supple, the chances are you will be healthy later on in life, enjoy the benefit of good vitality, stay mentally supple and feel young at heart. That should be a huge incentive for you to look after your joints and, fortunately, there are many ways of doing this.

Here are some interesting considerations about joints:

- You walk on water.

- Joints are reservoirs of fluid power.

- You move through life like your joints.

- Joints are the unofficial centres of the body.

- There's no need for arthritis (see page 68).

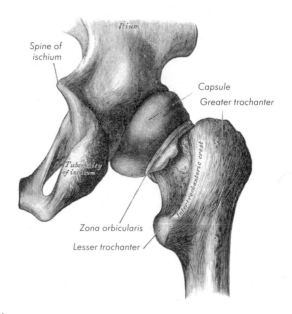

The hip joint

You walk on water

The next time you walk down the street, consider the fact that you are walking on water. Life is, after all, miraculous! All those joints of yours are filled with fluid. Bones don't actually touch each other, but are in relationship with other bones through joint fluid. Just that thought alone could completely change your whole relationship to your body! Just consider how many of these fluid spaces there are down the full length of your body. As you walk, your bones move through a fluid medium. So, the next time you walk down the street, see if you can appreciate this. It's an amazing feeling and can lead you to feeling light and fluid-like – more attuned to your true nature.

Joints are reservoirs of fluid power

Joints are filled with a special fluid secreted by the joint membrane, which makes the joint a hydraulic system. Dotted throughout you are, therefore, tiny reservoirs of fluid. In society, reservoirs are powerful resources and are essential for the maintenance of life. In the body, the joints are the body's reservoirs and are also places of power. It's worth sitting with that fact for a few minutes and contemplating it. Joints are places that feed the body, like reservoirs fuel our homes and industry. If you can really connect with that concept, then there's a tremendous source of power available to you which will last your whole life.

You move through life like your joints

In their very structure, joints are places of transition, adaptation and motion. Healthy joints create a natural ability to adapt and transform, to move with the flow of life. You can spot this in your life by noticing how well you adapt to new things. If you take things in your stride then you adapt well. Notice people around you. How well do they adapt? Notice, too, how mobile they are. Do they move with grace and fluidity? Generally, I've observed that people who are healthy and supple in their joints can flow with what life brings them and seem to have the ability to transform any given circumstance. When people are stiff and reflect poor mobility, they can display difficulty in adapting to new and changing events around them and flowing through life is generally problematic.

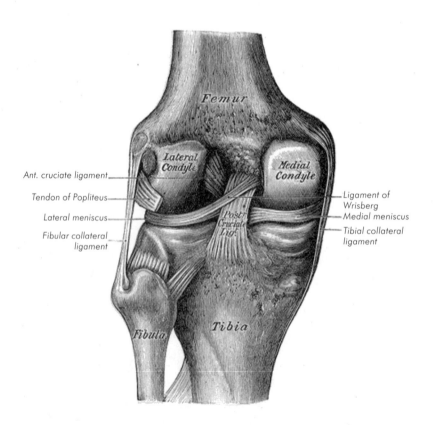

The knee joint

Physically, muscles attach or insert around joints. Arteries, veins, nerves and lymph vessels are all affected in their transition through joints. If joints are healthy, fluids and impulses move easily, but if they are fixed, dense or dehydrated, muscles have to work harder, impeding nerve impulses, fluid exchange and movement of blood. This leads to local stagnation, often painful or swollen joints, and if this persists, the whole body compensates, forcing other joints to become similarly affected. Over time the body becomes exhausted and painful and this could lead to even further disease. You get the idea of how much communication occurs through your joints!

Since they are so vibrant with communication, energy and potency, let's look at some ways to recognize and increase their health/consciousness and reap the rewards of fluid motion.

Exercise: Rejuvenating joints

Take a joint. Any joint. Let's say it's your knee – that's a joint that's often under a lot of strain and can feel unhappy. Here's a way to make it happier by breathing into it. Start by coming into a sense of your breath. Follow your breath for a while, with your attention, and then suspend your belief and imagine that air can descend down through the body beyond the lungs. See how that feels. It's a bit strange at first, but you'll notice your body respond. Imagine the breath descending slowly down through the pelvis and into the leg, so that eventually over a few minutes you are 'breathing' into your knee joint. Keep noticing small and subtle responses from your body. Stay with this for a while and notice how it affects your knee. Then change the image slightly by recognizing that you are taking air in from all around you into your knee joint. Making this slight shift is a way of connecting your knee to your whole body and the natural forces around it. Now see what your knee feels like. Once you are familiar with the signals from your body you can use this exercise to shift the state of any joint in your body – a useful tool to hold on to.

Joints are the unofficial centres of the body

It is often true that joints are experienced as places where things go wrong. Places that are weak and prone to giving trouble – resulting in pain and loss of movement. Here's a thought: what if we saw our joints for what they really are? *Joints are places of power and strength in the body, not places of weakness or fragility.* Think about all your joints as places of strength and vitality. Stand up still and feel how your body is divided into hundreds of joints, and it's the joints that make up the core of you. Imagine how each joint is connected to another joint through the bones. That's the reason why bones are called connective tissue. It's not the joints that are the connectors for bones, but bones are the connectors for joints. That's a big transition in belief and experience. It's also a quantum leap to change your perception of yourself from one of fragility to one of strength. See if you can shift the idea of yourself to one that sees your joints as the centres of your body. Your body is now organized around your joints, not around your brain or heart, gut or bones. The joints, as centres, connect all other parts of the body, bringing them all into communication. It's as if the joints are nodes for a computerized local area network.

There's no need for arthritis

Osteoarthritis is one of the most common illnesses in the modern world and many people suffer from painful joints in their later years. Why is this and is there any need for it? Osteoarthritis is inflammation of the joints, through wear and tear, and can be extremely painful and debilitating. Joints become swollen and lose their mobility, especially in the hands, hips, knees and parts of the spine. Contributing to arthritis is the increasing sedentary nature of our society and obesity. People have never moved their joints less than in the past 40 years, and the increase of weight on the body puts an extra burden on the joints. There's a simple solution. Keep your joints mobile through intelligent exercise (Chi Kung, Pilates and Alexander work, for instance) and keep them hydrated by drinking water. More importantly, perceive them according to their intrinsic nature and you'll learn how to avoid negative behaviours and instead encourage optimum health.

JOINT CITY

The hands and feet have quite a few joints: 28 in each hand and foot, making 112 joints in total. The limbs don't have a lot: 4 for each limb, making it 16 joints altogether. The head has 86, and the chest and throat area 28. So, that's already 246 joints. Now, as we know, the spine has numerous joints – 100 in fact. That means around a third of the joints in the body are all in the spine, making it highly flexible. So, there's as much flexibility in your spine as there is in your hands and feet. It's like a metropolis of joints!

The joints in the spine are different from the synovial joints, which are essentially bags of fluid. In the spine, the joints have flat disc-shaped structures in between them that have a tough outer ring, like a doughnut, with soft pulpy stuff in the middle, like jam. When the spine is healthy, the outer ring is strong and robust and holds in the jam, so that the jam acts like a ball bearing around which the two spinal vertebrae can easily move. This gives the spine the most wonderful ability to twist and turn and provides a cushioning along the whole length of the spine.

Exercise: Improving posture

Let's try and experience this aspect of our spines. As mentioned, the disc joints of the spine are like doughnuts with the centre acting like a ball bearing, so that the vertebral bones above and below them have freedom to move. Using this image, let's start with the top vertebrae of your spine and imagine them moving around these small ball bearings. Give your spine the opportunity to transform itself through the use of this image. You might notice it starts to feel more alive and even wants to glide more, as if it's had a sudden injection of oil. Be open to your spine improving its own alignment. Keep travelling down the spine a few vertebrae at a time. The exercise should take about 15 minutes. When you've worked through all the vertebrae, notice how your spine feels. Using this particular image connects you to the intrinsic nature of the spine and hence its natural purpose and quality, and serves as a reminder to the vast possibilities of movement throughout your spine. It is often too easy to forget, and even override, the natural flexibility of the spine in our busy daily lives. By repeating this exercise you will encourage your spine to remain flexible, and you may even discover that it maintains an intelligence of how to continue to move, and this feeling will spread throughout your body.

As you can imagine, restrictions in any area along the spine will affect function of target organs and, in particular, your posture. If your posture is poor, or you have an accident where the spine suffers a blow, then the joint weakens and the outer layer of the disk can struggle to hold in the jam and it starts to bulge. This causes pain by pressing on and irritating the nerves exiting from the spine. This, in turn, causes conditions like sciatica, or strange nerve symptoms such as tingling or numbness, and even referred pain, which reveals itself in other areas of the body and can be misleading. This is obviously not an ideal position to be in and living with such conditions for a long period of time exacerbates the problem. In such circumstances it's best to find appropriate treatment, but even better than this would be to have an understanding of what your spine actually feels like, in order for you to make appropriate interventions at earlier stages.

Exercise: Finding these joints

Let's use the breath to explore the nature of the joints in the spine. Follow your breath through your nose to the back of your mouth. This is just in front of the top of the spine. Imagine there's a portal into the top-most part of the spine and imagine your breath can move into the top joints of the spine. With each in-breath, follow your breath further into the spine. As you continue to breathe, let your breath move down the length of the spine. Your intention is to breathe into the large disc joints between each pair of vertebrae. Take your time. Let your breath descend through the spine in the neck and into the spine in the chest. How do the joints feel? Do you have a sense of them? As you go, you can self-assess your spinal joints. Some of them might feel healthy and vibrant, others might feel dense and difficult to breathe through. Some might feel like you are breathing into a large space. It's remarkable the spectrum of effects you can get. Carry on down the length of the entire spine. At the end, breathe along the length of all the joints and imagine you can breathe into the centres of the joints, the pulpy bit. What does it feel like? The whole exercise should take about 15 minutes. Trust your intuition and stay with areas that feel difficult to breathe through. By being able to breathe through the difficult areas you might notice some change occurring naturally in your spine.

Exercise: Fluid spine

One third of the structure of the spine is composed of fluid-filled joints, that is, a third of the height of the spine is joint, not bone. It means that your spine has a natural fluidity to it and, as such, you should be able to move from your core with fluid-like motion. So, let's consider the fluid nature of your spine. Standing still in the centre of a room, let your mind take in this aspect of yourself. Let it soak through you so that you come into the reality of it. Feel your spine's natural fluidity. Let it course through your whole body. Wait and encourage your body to move from its fluid spine in any way it wants. Don't try and predict it; keep a neutral attitude and let your mind be still and non-constraining. Just allow natural motion to emerge and unfold from your fluid spine. Don't get too earnest about it – have a sense of interest and amusement at what unfolds. Enjoy it.

The idea behind these exercises is for you to engage with them as often as possible, building up a good felt sense of the nature of your spine and developing a thorough understanding of its condition. This enables you to address any issues that appear more promptly, but also simply gives you the opportunity to enjoy the health within your spine.

A NOTE ON FLEXIBILITY/FLUIDITY

Suppleness varies tremendously in people due to inherited factors and body type. If you experience yourself as not being supple, it doesn't necessarily mean you're unhealthy. So don't worry if you can't bend yourself in all directions. The important thing is that you optimize your health so you become as supple as you can. The thing to avoid is stiffness, pain, and lack of movement and flexibility in joints.

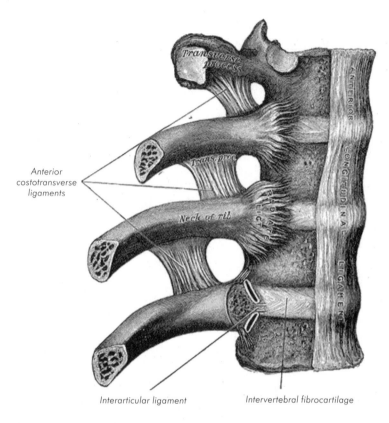

Anterior costotransverse ligaments

Interarticular ligament

Intervertebral fibrocartilage

The costovertebral joints (joining the ribs to the spinal column)

PARTICULARLY AMAZING JOINTS

It's really easy to get lost in the multitude of joints along the spine and forget that there are some other particularly significant joints in the body. These joints are so significant that they affect the health of the whole body. They are found at the top of the spine, bottom of the spine and the joint at the jaw. They're the big three! If these three joints are happy, then you will live a long and healthy life. It really is that simple. In fact, if you didn't bother too much about anything else, but made sure these three places were balanced and not under strain, you would be doing well. Your posture will be optimal, as will your breath, your nervous system will be able to move easily between active and relaxed states, etc. – the list goes on. You could make it even simpler and say that if the jaw joint and the joints at the top of the spine are healthy, then the bottom of the spine will sort itself out. So concentrate on your jaw and neck for optimal health.

Top of the spine

Do you find yourself constantly trying to relax your neck? Does it feel like your shoulders are pulling your head down? Does your neck crunch when you move it? Or, do you feel like your neck is twisted or bent? If you can answer yes to any of these questions, then you almost certainly have strain at the top two joints of the spine, pictured below. These joints are critical to the

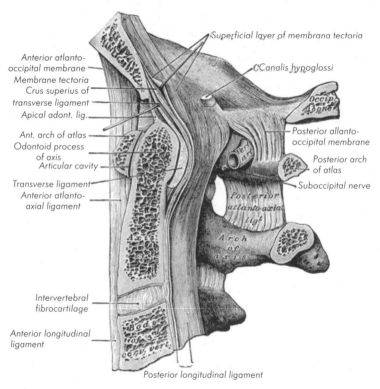

The top of the spine

balance of your whole body. They take the weight of the head (no small thing) and ideally translate it in a straight line down the spine. The head is a heavy object that constantly needs to move and reposition itself to talk, eat and sense, and that is a tall order for the body. Most of the strain is taken by two of the smallest joints of the spine. They connect the bottom of the skull with the first bone of the spine (tilting of the head) and the first bone with the second bone of the spine (rotating of the head). The first bone is called the atlas, because it supports the world that is the head. The second is called the axis, because it is the axis for the turning of the head. The health of these two joints affects your whole body. This is such a critical place for muscles, nerves and blood flow and how your head relates to your body. How do you feel this place is in you?

Bottom of the spine

The old axiom 'as above so below' or even 'as below so above' is certainly true of the spine. The ends definitely mimic each other. Neck tension will equal lower back tension. Strain in the top two joints equals strain in the lower two joints. The reason for this is that all the weight of the upper body passes through the lowest joints of the spine. Not surprisingly most people have pain and discomfort here and a lack of mobility. The key structure is the bone called the sacrum (see the picture on the next page). This is the bottom of the spine and the back of the pelvis. It's a triangular bone that has three joints. There's a joint at the top of the triangular shape (the sacrum) that meets the last vertebral disk of the spine (the lumbo-sacral joint) and then two joints along either side of the triangular bone meeting the bones of the pelvis (sacro-iliac joints). The relationship at the top of the spine is like a pivot, whereas at the bottom of the spine it's a triangle of forces. How do you feel this area is in you? Do you get a sense of any similarity to what's going on at the top of your spine?

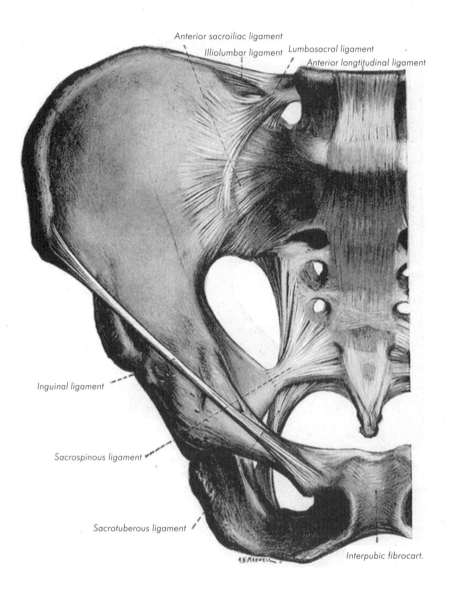

Anterior sacroiliac ligament

Illiolumbar ligament   Lumbosacral ligament

Anterior longtitudinal ligament

Inguinal ligament

Sacrospinous ligament

Sacrotuberous ligament

Interpubic fibrocart.

The bottom of the spine

The jaw

The jaw may not seem an obvious place to be of such importance, but if you look at people's jaws you will notice many
things. First, how tense they can be. This is one of the tensest
places on the earth, maybe even the universe. Lots of our tension about life goes into the jaw. Fear, anger and grief can all be
held in the chewing muscles. This is where we do our emotional
repression. Anatomically, the joint becomes compressed, and
our head starts to tighten up through constant muscle tension.
Often, this leads to headaches and poor fluid exchange. Teeth
become unhappy, the eyes start to feel like there's suddenly no
room to move in their sockets, sinuses start to feel small and
compressed, the mucous membranes tighten and there's an increase in mucus production. The worst consequence, though, is
that the top of the neck starts to tense up too, and that affects
the whole spine and therefore the whole body. So how you

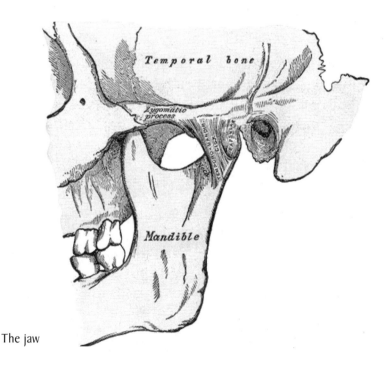

The jaw

walk and your posture will be affected. Many strange symptoms can relate back to a tight jaw. TMJ (temporomandibular joint) syndrome has become a medically accepted fact. Along with jaw tension comes pelvic floor tension and diaphragm tension affecting your digestion and breathing. They all seem to go hand in hand. That's all a bit of a nightmare scenario, I know, so let's not dwell on it too long. Just to say if you've got jaw tension it will definitely be affecting other places in your body.

Try the following jaw tests:

- *Look in a mirror.* See what your jaw looks like. Have a good look at it. Look at it in comparison with your head and neck. Does it look tense or relaxed? If it's tense, there's often a look of the whole face being squished and your eyes starting slightly. If your face is relaxed the jaw looks like it's just hanging there. Check too if there's an orientation to the left or right. That might be to do with tension on one side of the jaw. Or if it is jutting forwards, which can be to do with some tensions in specific muscles.

- *How wide can you open it?* Put your hand into a fist. Point the knuckles at your mouth and see how many you can put between your teeth. Three knuckles is healthy and normal, two knuckles means it's tight, one knuckle means you've got lock-jaw, four knuckles means you're an anaconda!

- *Signs of jaw tension.* If you like to chew a lot of gum or grind your teeth at night you will be doing this because your jaw is tight. Notice if you catch yourself gritting your teeth unconsciously. Half the time you may not even realize your jaw is constantly tight.

- *Feel the chewing muscles.* Put your hands over your temples and tighten your jaw. You should feel muscles bunching up. These are the temporalis muscles and they attach to the top of the jaw and radiate through the temples right up to the sides of the head above the ear. Is one tighter than the other? When these muscles are constantly tense, they clamp the head and you can feel as if your head is in a vice, which often brings on a headache. The other major chewing muscle is around the angle of the jaw. Follow the jaw back from your chin till the bone changes angles and starts to move up rather than back. Feel on the sides of the jaw around the angle. If these muscles are tight it will be sore. They are called the masseters and are thick and solid and more obviously give the jaw the appearance of being clenched. These are the ones that cartoonists exaggerate.

- *Feel the TMJ.* This stands for temporomandibular joint, which means ear-jaw joint. You can find it by bringing the tip of one of your fingers in front of each ear. Move the finger around and up and down in front of it until you find a depression. When you think you've got it, open and close your jaw and you should feel the joint moving. How do the joints feel? Do they glide when they open or do they feel sticky and resistant?

- *What happens when you clench it?* Tighten your jaw and notice what else in your body tightens. This can highlight interesting correspondences like your pelvic floor tightens up or you feel your breathing tenses and holds, or your lower back tightens too. Do it a few times so that you can get a real sense of repercussions.

Exercise: How to relax the jaw

If your jaw has been tense for a long time it's not especially easy to relax it. And a long time might be from anything up to many years. Here's an attempt. Let your jaw hang open as much as you can so that your mouth gapes open. Imagine the jaw is heavy. Don't use any muscles to do this. At first it will feel silly, but as you stay with it you will notice there is an initial relaxing and then you will notice particular areas of tension. These tend to be the chewing muscles. Notice where the tension is located, then imagine that the tension is dissolving. You can use any image for this. A common one is ice melting, or just imagine the muscle is melting. Stay with it for a while longer. Keep doing the exercise a few times a day and your jaw will let go and feel freer. As it does this, notice any changes that take place in your body other than in the jaw itself – your heart may feel calmer, your breathing may become deeper, and certain aches and pains in your head or spine might well dissolve too. How does your jaw feel now? Are you talking differently? Notice how you relate to people now – has this changed? Are you feeling more confident or outgoing? Do you view the world around you differently? Do the exercise over a period of three days and make a note of changes at the end of each day.

Who's ever heard of the sternoclavicular joint?

It's hard to talk about the top joints in the spine and the jaw without mentioning the sternoclavicular joints. Few people have ever heard of the sternoclavicular joints other than, say, anatomists, yet they are fascinating and important joints to remember, as they are the only joints that connect your arms to your trunk (i.e. where the arms meet the body). Considering their purpose, they're not very big – little things at the top of the chest, for us all to see. You can feel them by using your fingertips: contact the centre of the chest, move your fingers up to the top of the chest meeting the bottom of the neck, where you will find the small bony protrusions of the sternoclavicular joints. Keep your fingers there and move your arms around in a circular motion, a bit like a chicken, and you should feel the joints glide.

HOW PROFOUND ARE YOUR JOINTS?

Joints and time (being in the present)

Motion is the ability to be adaptive, sensitive and in the moment. Your joints are in a constant process of evaluation. In order to move, you have to be able to find the centre-point between forward and backward movements, creating a balanced state between past and future so that you can move in the present. How many times have you slowed down in order to recall something in your thoughts, or sped up to rush ahead to an appointment? With this in mind, how many people actually move in the present? Just observe yourself and others and see how your movements are caught up either in the past or in the future. Especially observe the knees – how many people lock their knees? Try doing this and notice how it feels. Many people have the opposite occurring in their knees too, constantly in a flexed position, as if they're about to run. Again put your knees in this position and notice how it feels. Now try to find a balanced state between these two extremes. What does this do to your state?

Being joined (being in relationship)

Joints allow your body to communicate and bring into relationship all its separate parts. This is a microcosm of how you relate in your life. Building healthy relationships comes from healthy internal relationships. As your joints change and become more

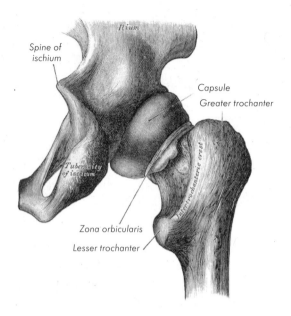

mobile through the exercises in this chapter, observe how you relate to other people. The healthier and more connected your internal relationships are, the more natural, confident and authentic you become in the world.

Joints make the world go round (being in harmony)

You respond to the world around you through your joints by constantly adapting to your environment. Much of the nervous system is taken up with monitoring and responding to subtle changes around all the joint positions. This means that your joint position is in direct response to your environment. It's the reason why you can close your eyes, move your arms around, and still know where they're positioned in relation to the space around you. Our daily environment directly affects our joints, how we move and how we hold our posture. So choose your environment carefully. If the environment you live in is harmonious, then your joints will be healthy. Environments in which you feel threatened make your body tighten up, which means muscles and tendons are taut, creating strain in the joints, and fluids become unable to exchange easily. A powerful practice is to broaden out to the natural forces around you and let your body be affected by that deeper life rhythm. There's a natural harmony and order in these forces that allows your body to adjust to a deeper health. In this relationship, your joints are being informed by a more universal force that allows for greater connectivity.

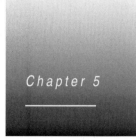

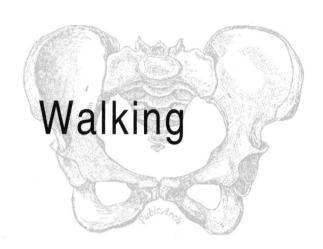

Chapter 5

Walking

Here's something we do a lot of the time. Just like breathing and eating. We walk, and we take it for granted. You only recognize how important it is when you can't do it. Try recuperating from a leg injury and you'll soon realize how complex walking is. Vast tracts of the brain are involved in the coordination of your body's movements, particularly those involving your legs and hands such as walking and manipulating objects. The enlarged brain evolved just to cope with the demands of walking on two legs. Even though you might not be consciously occupied with the mechanics of walking, your brain, nervous system and a large part of your body are definitely highly involved with it. Like breathing, it all shifts into the background to leave you free to think.

Walking is a big thing in your life and a large part of your vitality is used for it. Once you start to connect with all the elements involved in it, you can transform your walking to be more efficient and gain a balanced posture. You'd be surprised by how much energy people lose from inefficient walking. You can change this by getting to know how you walk. Feel how you walk. When you start to be more present with the muscles and nerves involved, you can then adjust your body's processes and move through life in a different way. Below are several exercises to help you with this.

Exercise: Walking around

The fact that we are bipedal and walk upright is greatly underestimated. Try walking around the room slowly, concentrating only on how you move. See if you can feel the nuances of every step. Can you feel all the different muscle movements? Walk even slower, as if in slow motion. Can you feel the adjustments in your breath, posture, spine as well as the angle of your head as you walk? How many thousands of individual movements are involved in a single step? Keep practising this and you will develop a natural understanding of your body's way of moving that will leave you in awe.

Exercise: Have you heard of the psoas?

The major muscles for walking are located deep in the lower back and pelvis. They are called the psoas muscles. You can feel them by placing your hand on your lower back and walking round the room. Pay particular attention to how much contraction is occurring there. Every time your leg steps forward the psoas muscle contracts and pulls the leg forward, anchoring from the lower spine. Your legs are big limbs, so the psoas is a really large and long muscle. Keep walking and you'll soon notice that you walk from your lower spine. Now place your hands on the front of your abdomen, under your navel. What happens when you walk? Can you feel any contraction here? It's often hard to feel any contraction here as these muscles are commonly so weak.

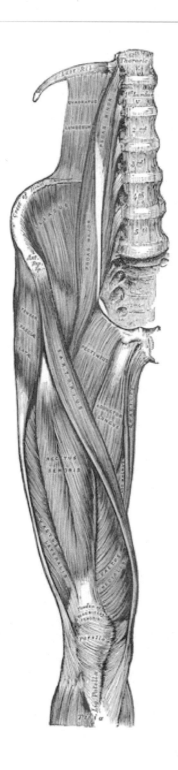

Thigh muscles

Place your hands on the very top part of your thighs, so that you don't have to bend forwards and change the way you walk. How much do these muscles tighten? Listen to your buttocks too! There are also muscles here that participate in walking. The other relevant muscles are in the lower legs and help flex the knees and ankles. Spend time being aware of these muscles too, especially in the calves and along the front of your lower legs. It takes time to get to know your body and how it works. Spend time listening and learning from your body and you'll discover a whole meditation and contemplation around the simple act of walking. If repeated often enough, you will be truly amazed by the intricacy of walking and the clarity of perception you can develop.

Exercise: Walking from the spine

When you walk, the whole body is involved in maintaining your uprightness and this especially implicates the muscles along the spine. You can perceive them almost like a tram track up the length of the spine. They tense as you walk. Try feeling this by placing the palm of your hand on the back of your neck. As you walk, you will feel the intricacy of the muscles involved in the neck, as they seek to maintain upper body and head stability, subtly compensating for the lower body movements. Stay with this for a while as it will take some getting used to. Over time, you will start to get a deeper and clearer experience of how you move. Now tune into the bottom of the spine by touching the sacrum, and feel how you move from here. This gives you an interesting comparison of how different the movements are in the sacrum from in the neck. It would be good to consider whether your whole spine moves in response to walking. Does your whole body move? Are there areas that don't? What do these areas feel like?

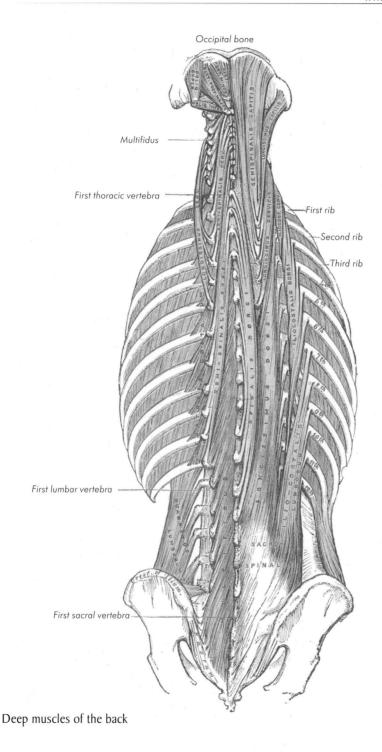

Occipital bone

Multifidus

First thoracic vertebra

First rib

Second rib

Third rib

First lumbar vertebra

First sacral vertebra

Deep muscles of the back

Exercise: Walking with your spine

Imagine that your spine is in the space in front of you. Place one hand so that the fingers wrap around the top of the spine and the other hand wraps around the lumbar spine. Walk with your hands in these positions in front of you reflecting and mimicking the length of the spine. Walk slowly. Stay with the image of the spine. While you're walking, turn slightly to the right and left, following what happens in your spine as you do this – notice how it rotates in the two areas you are focused on and how there is a change in curvature. This is a way of tuning in to your spine, resonating with how your spine moves and also with the energetic dynamics of it. Notice how your body moves from your spine.

Now imagine that your breath can move down the length of your spine. Be open to breathing into your spine around the top hand and then allow it to descend to the bottom hand. This should bring more awareness of how your spine moves. After a while try synchronizing your breath with your walk. Breathe in down the spine when you bring your leg up to step, and breathe out when you shift your weight into your leg as you step. Move slowly, let your balance have time to adjust as you shift your centre of gravity in the walk. Staying with your natural breath should slow your walking down. The main thing is to appreciate how your spine is the central axis for all movement. Notice when you truly move from this axis, what that feels like and how your state of mind is when you do this. Compare that to when you are moving off this axis and how it feels and what happens to your state of mind.

ONE STEP – THE ANATOMY OF WALKING

Taking one step involves a symphony of neuro-muscular activity way beyond our imagination. As you become more sensitive to these activities, your body will automatically adjust to an optimal movement. It requires only conscious awareness to be able to start changing.

Let's feel exactly what's involved in just one step:

- A step starts with the psoas muscle tightening to bring the leg through in front of you.

- Then, the muscles of the thigh tighten, along with muscles in the abdomen, to bring the leg upwards.

- Next, the muscles at the front of your lower leg tighten in order to position the foot accurately on the ground. Your heel will be the first part of the foot to touch the ground.

- You then have to push forward for the next step and you'll feel your calves having to tighten, as well as your hamstrings, and your weight has to shift into the balls of your feet.

- Whilst all this is happening, there are many muscles in the feet that tense to keep the angle of the foot correct and to stabilize the ankle joint.

When you slow the step down, you will easily notice all of these movements as they become exaggerated, because the muscles have to work harder in order to fulfil the step. Become aware of the parts of the step that you are particularly drawn to. Walking in this way will highlight how you step and what muscles are strong or weak. It may be that a step is difficult for your body to make on one side – try to slow this part of the step down so that you can feel what is happening. It could be that you need to strengthen some of your muscles to improve this, or adjust your balance. Perhaps you aren't moving from the centre of your pelvis or spine or maybe it's to do with your whole body alignment.

Exercise: Walking from your guts

Bring your awareness into your abdominal muscles. You can spread your hands across them and notice how much activity there is as you walk. Move your hands on to the sides of your waist and notice what's happening as you move. You should be able to feel the muscles tensing underneath your hands. Make a note of how much they tighten. If you do not have a strong sense of your muscles tensing in your abdomen, then your muscles in your lower back will be working too hard. If you notice that one side of your waist is tighter than the other, then that could lead to your posture being out of alignment. Try to deepen your awareness into your guts that lie beneath the muscles of the abdomen. Imagine walking from this place! Connect to a deep place in your guts, just underneath your umbilicus, and see how this changes your walk. Once you shift your attention to feel how you walk from your guts, you may notice what a crucial role they play in the act of walking and how, once engaged properly, they contribute to good posture.

Exercise: Where is your centre of gravity?

To discover your centre of gravity, stand with your legs shoulder-width apart and place your palms in front of your pelvis at the place you found in your guts. Slowly shift your weight into your left leg and step forward with your right leg, heel touching the floor first and then allowing your body weight to spread evenly and smoothly throughout the length of the whole foot. Make sure you spread your foot as it makes contact with the floor. As you walk, allow your belly to soften so that your breathing can subtly swell the abdomen. Breathe in as you draw your leg up, and breathe out as you place it on the ground and shift your weight forward. Pay attention to how it feels to move from your pelvis and how the pelvis is like your centre of gravity for walking.

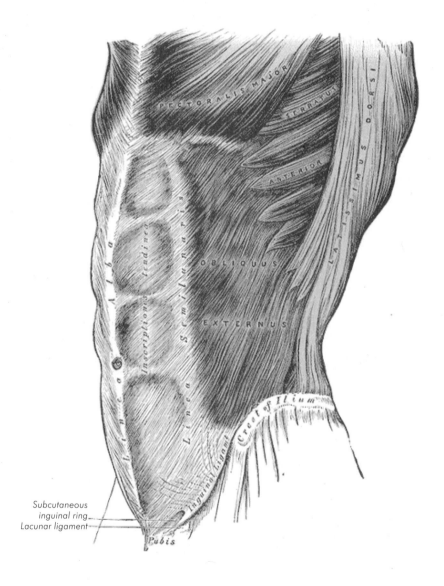

Subcutaneous
inguinal ring
Lacunar ligament

External oblique muscle of the abdomen

Another way to experience your pelvis as the centre of gravity is, on the in-breath, to let your hands move off the surface of your abdomen and out into the space at the sides of the pelvis and, on the out-breath, to bring your hands back in to the centre of your pelvis. See if you can have a sense of expansion and contraction from the centre of your pelvis. When you move your hands out, keep them at the same level to the centre of your pelvis. Let your palms look forwards in front of you. Practise this until you become confident. This exercise is a powerful way of creating awareness of the space that immediately surrounds you and, at the same time, of your internal space within your body.

As a further variation on the theme, try letting your hand position gradually move up the length of the body. Start with the above exercise then, when you breathe in, move your hands out from the centre of your pelvis and up to the level of your umbilicus and, on the out-breath, move them back down to the pelvis. Once you've stayed with that for a while, move your hands higher up to the level of your diaphragm and see what that does for you. In a similar way, bring your hands up to the level of your chest, shoulders and head, always making a connection back to the pelvis with each out-breath. These movements will give you an insight into how your body moves from different places within it, how it coordinates breathing and movement and how you orientate yourself in space. It breaks down the elements of walking into small bits. Remember, all of these elements are occurring automatically as you walk. Becoming more conscious of them will allow you to change how you walk in space and that, in turn, will change how you walk through life.

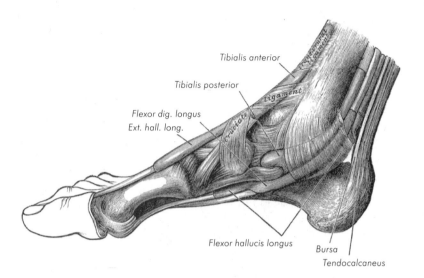

Tibialis anterior

Tibialis posterior

Flexor dig. longus
Ext. hall. long.

Flexor hallucis longus

Bursa

Tendocalcaneus

Exercise: Walking with your feet on the ground

Many of us walk with our feet barely touching the ground. It could
be from walking too fast, so that there's little time spent on our
heels, or through poor posture, so that only the edge or a small
part of the surface area of the foot is in contact with the ground.
Check if you are doing this. You might be living your life on the
balls of your feet. Sometimes this can be caused by your pelvic
floor being too tight – check if it is. Sit for a few minutes on a chair
and bring your awareness to your pelvic floor. It's composed of
a number of muscles running from front to back and across the
pelvis. Let it relax by inviting it to relax mentally. Invite your pelvic
floor to sink into the seat of the chair. Allow all the structures
around the pelvic floor to relax, especially the area around your
groin, at the top of both legs, and your buttocks, at the back of
your pelvis. We commonly carry tension in the pelvic floor that
we have become so accustomed to that we no longer register it.

It can often be to do with tensions in other areas of the body. So let your shoulders and diaphragm relax too. These two structures greatly influence the pelvic floor. As you relax your shoulders and diaphragm is there a difference in your pelvic floor? Now stand and walk around the room. Do you walk differently with a relaxed pelvic floor? It can feel profoundly different as if you are sinking into your legs more.

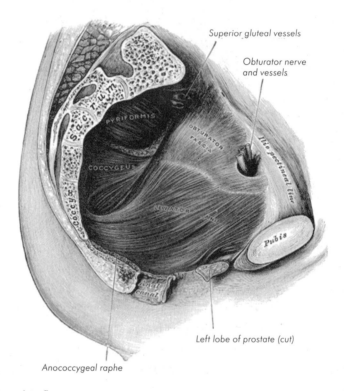

Superior gluteal vessels

Obturator nerve and vessels

Left lobe of prostate (cut)

Anococcygeal raphe

The pelvic floor

Now try to relax your feet. A good way to do this is to have some reflexology or to massage your feet yourself. Find a seat and spend a few minutes loosening up your foot by the ankle, between the webbing of the toes, the arch of the foot and the sole by shaking, slapping and using your thumbs to press. When you've completed this, see how it feels to stand and walk. This time round it should feel like your feet widen as you step on to them and as if you're sinking into the ground. With this feeling comes quite a different state of awareness of your body and your mind will operate differently.

WALKING FROM THE EARTH/ WALKING WITH THE EARTH

There's a natural spring in the earth that can feel like a rising force if you get in touch with it. When you walk, and really allow your step to sink into the earth, you will feel a lift that buoys you up in your stride and brings about a natural energizing of your whole body, particularly in the spine. In this way, walking becomes revitalizing and not an effort. It means that as you walk you can be in a different relationship with the earth. Be open to this. Give yourself the time to bring a new awareness to walking and to your body. Your walking can deepen into a much richer phenomenon that brings you in touch with nature and soil. Soil cultivates growth, and you can be fed by it too. Walking with this kind of attention will connect you to being part of the planet, not separate from it. Your whole body will start to relate to the earth and your guts and organs will become earthy. It also helps the brain earth its electrical charge. As a result your mind becomes quieter and you become increasingly sensitive to the natural world around you, all from just changing how you walk!

WALKING WITH THE UNIVERSE

We walk upright with the ground under our feet and the sky above our heads – between heaven and earth. Beyond the sky is the universe. As you are open to the earth below, try being open to the sky above, bringing the universal into your walk. The natural spring from the earth will make you interested in the space beyond you. It opens you up to the inspiration of the universe we live in, so that the next time you walk down the street you are in a very different relationship to your environment. It's no longer about what's going on in your head or about the immediacy of your particular life, but more about what's going on in your body, around your body, underneath you and above you. It's about balancing the everydayness of life with the greatness of life. It's about bringing the universal into your life. So spend time understanding how you walk so that you can have the whole of the universe supporting you.

Chapter 6

Blood

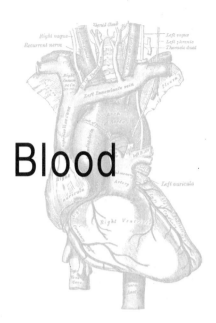

Find a quiet place and sit still for a while so that you can listen to your body. The first thing you should notice is your breathing, then see if you can slowly filter that out. The best way to do this is simply to get used to it being there, then you can concentrate on feeling the next biggest movement, the beating of the heart. Once you become fully aware of it, it can feel like the whole body shudders each time there's a heartbeat, especially in the upper body. As you sit listening to the movements of the heart, notice what your reaction is. For some people a feeling of alarm can emerge, for fear of the heart stopping. If this arises in you just recognize your response and acknowledge it. See if you can allow this alarm to settle so that you can bring your attention to noticing the health of your heart and how powerful it is. After all, it's the most powerful muscle in the body and has been beating since you were an embryo. Why doubt its powers now? The heart can often be depicted as a soft, gentle, fragile organ that can break, when in reality, it's quite the opposite. It's tough, strong and robust, so no need to fear. This is your strongest organ made of the toughest tissue in the body – cardiac muscle tissue. It's much denser and stronger than normal muscle. Plus, it's got its own neural network that is separate from the brain, the 'heart brain' – an intrinsic nervous conduction system that paces the heart's contractions. So now you know the heart is both powerful and intelligent. Sit with that fact for a while and allow it to echo through your body and mind. Give your mind and body a chance to accept and absorb this, and let go of fear.

Now bring your hands to the area of the heart so that you can feel it directly. It occupies most of the middle area of the chest and to the left of the centre. It's about the size of your fisted hand. As you follow its beat you might notice the movement of the diaphragm right underneath it. The heart sits on the middle of the diaphragm and is moved by its contraction and relaxation during breathing. The diaphragm, in turn, along with the other structures in the area, is also moved by the beating of the heart. See if you can feel both of these movements, influencing each other and the other organs in the area. Between them they create a lot of internal movement – the body is not a quiet place.

RIVERS OF BLOOD

The next big movement to notice is the gushing of blood. Incredibly, it's not so obvious even though 7–8 pints of red fluid is constantly moving through the body. The heart pumps 20 gallons of blood a day! We've got a river of blood roaring through us – a waterfall flowing into all the body's tissues and cells. That's not so easy to imagine, so take your time with the images. Let the images bring you into the feelings of blood movement. Once you get it, it can feel exhilarating.

INSIDE WE ARE RED

Inside we are bright red and deep red, like vermillion. That's our most abundant colour – much more abundant than the colour of our skin. So we are the same colour after all, and yet none of us remember that. Instead, we notice the obvious, the superficial, not what lies beneath. It's a shame really, because therein lies most of our true common ground, as humans and as animals, that we could celebrate.

Exercise: Heart and hands

Sitting still in a quiet room, come into a sense of your heart again. Be with the beat of it for a while and then open up to the possibility of feeling movement of fluid through it. The heart has two sets of double chambers – one on the right and one on the left. The right is for receiving blood from the entire body and the left is for sending blood back to the whole body. The heart is so powerful that the blood vessels coming off the left side need to be very thick and robust to withstand the pressure. These vessels are called arteries and they are wrapped in smooth muscle that can contract and relax like normal muscles. Let's follow the flow of blood out of the left chambers. This vessel is called the aorta and it moves directly up and then forms an arch to the left, before it travels down and arches in behind the heart in front of the spine (deep in the chest), then descends through the diaphragm into the abdomen. Off the arch are the major arteries for the head and arms. You can follow the flow of blood into the arch and out to the arms and hands. See if you can feel a flow moving up from the heart and out through the shoulders and arms. It's like a river running to your hands. If you follow it you can feel a constant flow into the hands. Realize that your heart is supplying blood to your hands enabling you to do all the things you do with your hands – which is most of what we do, so your heart is always connected to your hands. That's a profound image. Let that sink in for a while and notice what ideas or insights emerge.

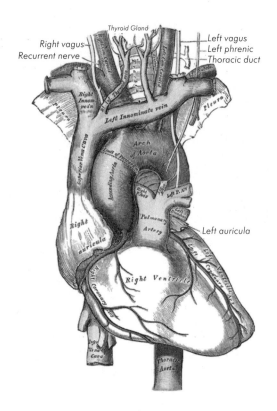

The heart

HEART FEEDS THE BRAIN

There's a similar movement occurring with the flow of blood to the head through the carotid arteries, except it's much more powerful, more like a raging torrent. The brain is hungry for blood all the time and it requires a full, constant, strong flow. Try following the blood flow in the neck. The arteries are kept deep within the neck and they then divide at the top of the neck into an internal and an external branch. You might even feel this in yourself. Part of the blood flow goes externally to the head and face and the internal branch moves into the interior of the head through little holes in the bones of the floor of the cranium. There is one hole either side as there are two carotids, on the left and right sides of the neck. When the vessel enters what is essentially the bottom of the brain, it forms a circle that acts like a main ring of blood for the whole brain. Many other arteries fan out from this ring taking blood into all parts of the brain. From the heart you should be able to feel the flow of blood, up either side of the neck, through the bony base of the cranium, into the Circle of Willis, and then emanating out from there to all parts of the brain. Be with that for a while. This is one of the ways your heart and brain are linked. It can feel like the heart is feeding the brain.

BLOOD CENTRE LINE

If you now follow your flow of blood up over the arch and down the aorta, in the centre of your chest, you can feel the strongest flow of blood in your body. Can you sense this? Seeing its shape in the image of the heart may help you feel it more strongly inside you. Notice how big it is – it's so big you can't really miss it. Sit still and be open to feeling this vital structure and the surge of blood moving through it. It's strong and powerful. As it descends through the body there are many branches feeding the organs, muscles and bones from it. Notice it moving through the diaphragm where a big hole has been created for it to pass through. It travels deep in the body for protection. Being one of your most vital structures, it's held just in front of the spine and it's from here that it can heat up the whole body – from the core of the torso.

As the aorta descends into the abdomen there are many branches feeding the organs and as it approaches the navel it branches into two, each branch feeding a leg with fresh blood. See if you can feel the crossroads. It's a significant place. Stay with the movement of one flow into two. The branches pass deep in each groin and move down the length of the leg to the feet. Just like with the hands, see if you can feel the connection between the heart, the aorta and the feet. If you feel that relationship it can be very grounding. It's like connecting to your feet through a fluid flow. Here's a deep and secret relationship: the feet are always connected to the heart.

THE HEART FEEDS ITSELF

Another important vessel to understand is the one that feeds the heart itself with blood. This is called the coronary artery and, as you know, it can fill up with fatty deposits and become constricted, producing angina, or it can function magnificently, bringing fresh blood (the freshest as it's the first branch off the aortic arch) continuously to your heart for the whole of your life. That's what it does most of the time. It's important to recognize that actually our bodies function well most of the time. Overall the heart rarely becomes ill or dysfunctional. Considering that the world's longevity is increasing, it's a remarkable task to achieve – respect to the heart.

SELF-DIAGNOSIS

It is possible that whilst you've been sensing your blood flowing through your arteries you may have had a sense of constriction. When you feel stressed or subject to high blood pressure, the nervous system will tell your major arteries to contract, thereby forcing the blood to move faster. If this persists it creates hypertension. This is an increasingly common condition and has degrees of expression. Check out how laid back or uptight you are by sensing into your aorta and heart. Does your heart feel that it's labouring or speeding? Or is it purring, like a well tuned, idling engine? Does your aorta feel tight or relaxed? You don't need instruments to measure these things – just listen to your body and self-assess. Finding your levels of stress and hypertension gives vital information on how to lead your life.

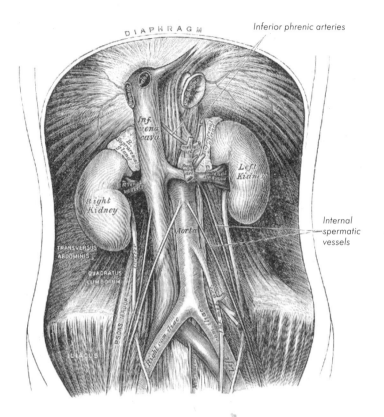

The abdominal aorta

THE GREAT RETURN

Once blood has reached the tissues of the body, it returns in vessels called veins. These are not as thick as arteries and have valves in them to stop the backflow of blood. The power generated by the heart is reduced in the veins and so blood return is encouraged by muscular movement and, in particular, by breathing, through the action of the diaphragm. The main highway up the body is the vena cava. It comes up the body on the right of the aorta. See if you can feel it pulsing. It's wider than the aorta. Follow your diaphragm at the same time as the vena cava. You can feel the diaphragm drawing blood up, acting like a pump. The vena cava returns blood from the whole body back to the heart into the right chamber.

CENTRE TO THE PERIPHERY – A UNIVERSAL MOTION

So, fresh oxygenated blood moves up and to the left before moving down the centre of the torso. Appreciate the movement of blood out from the centre of the chest to the extremities of the hands and fingers. Moving out and gathering back. Out from the aorta in the abdomen to the toes and feet. Appreciate the movement back. It's slower. It's got a different feel to it. The blood is different – it's deeper red. From thousands of tributaries a great river is formed that moves up the right side of the torso returning to the heart. Sit with this for a while; feel the ebb and flow of blood through the whole body, moving out to the periphery and back to the centre of the heart. This is a deep intrinsic movement of nature and the universe, a flowing out and then returning to a centre or source. It's like a pulse, an oscillating tide. It affects us deeply, creating a subtle consciousness that links us to many natural movements around us. Our blood flow intrinsically mirrors and connects us to the profound and inherent movements of the universe, right here in our own body, not out there in deep space or within the microcosm of the atom or an equation of physics. Sit and contemplate this for a while and see what thoughts and feelings emerge for you – what secrets of the universe unfold.

BLOOD IS POWER

A lot of people are afraid of blood, rather than the heart, because of bleeding. After all, blood is only seen when something has gone wrong, when the boundary of our skin has been penetrated, either by an accident or if someone is dying (i.e. a traumatic incident). Let's try to change the association and bring about a more enlightened relationship with blood. Think about what blood really is. Blood is food. It's what all your cells want beyond anything else. Blood is our ultimate nourishment – it's the real food for the body tissues and contains the raw materials for keeping your cells alive and for creating energy. Blood contains our vitality. Blood is life and often when we bleed it's described as our life force ebbing away. *Being conscious of the presence of blood within the body creates a direct link to your vitality.* The purpose of the above exercises is to encourage this link between your blood and your vitality. However, there are significant places of power that will bring you into a particularly strong link to this energy process within you. These are at the blood interfaces (or exchange sites) – the interface to the outside world through the lungs and gut (air and food), and the interface to the hormonal glands, as well as the interface to the inside world at a cellular level.

To help with the sense of these interfaces we'll use another image from nature. So far we've had rivers, waterfalls and ring flows, and now we find estuaries. These are the places where blood meets cells, at the ends of the arteries. The arteries split and split into finer and finer vessels, smaller and smaller and thinner and thinner, until they form web-like structures called capillary beds that look like estuaries or river deltas. There are billions of these in the body. As they are so thin (one cell thick), part of the blood can move out easily into the space between the capillaries and the cells. This is called the interstitial space and is the fluid space in which all cells reside and where exchange takes place. Hormones, oxygen and sugar are amongst the most common ingredients that are exchanged here. Wherever there are cells there are capillaries, because cells need a continuous supply of blood to live. Below are a couple of exercises for relating to the interface at the lungs and the interface at a cellular level (the interface at the gut will be explored in Chapter 10).

As previously mentioned in Chapter 3, the lungs are like bunches of grapes with the pulp taken out. Lots of little grape-shaped pockets called alveoli. Each of these has a web of capillaries woven around it. Blood from the heart comes into the capillary bed, there is a mixing with the air (oxygen in, carbon dioxide out) and the new blood moves through the other side of the bed and back to the heart to be taken into the aorta and out to the rest of the body. There are about 150 million alveoli per lung and each has its own capillary network. That's a terrific exchange!

Exercise: Blood meets air

Follow your breath with your attention. Notice how the air feels moving through your nose, throat and airways down into the lungs. See if you can feel the air enter your lungs. How does it feel? Can you feel the sensations of the air as it comes into the lungs? Stay with this feeling. You might distinguish between sensations at the top of your lungs and at the bottom. Maybe you can get a sense of the main pathways the air moves through. These are the bronchi and are shaped like branches of a tree. They feel quite distinctly firm as they contain rings of cartilage. Less distinct are the alveoli positioned all around them. They feel softer and more fluid-like. This is where air and blood meet. Examine this place for a while by feeling it. This is a powerful interface between two mediums. Maybe some of the sensations you feel are created by the diffusion of gas in the alveoli? Can you feel the energy of this? It can feel like you are drawing in energy from around you.

On the other side of the alveoli is a stream of blood from the heart flowing through the pulmonary capillaries. Be open to noticing the blood flow from the heart to the lungs. When it enters the lungs it slows as it meets the capillaries. It slows down in order to allow time for diffusion of gases. Blood returning from the lungs is now clearly different – it's oxygenated, bright red and feels more vibrant.

Now allow your awareness of the sensations and spaces in the lungs and the movement of blood through the capillaries to merge together. How does it all feel?

Exercise: Blood meets cells

There is a deeper kind of respiration that occurs at the other end of the blood system to the lungs. It's more of an internal one, where oxygen moves into the cells and carbon dioxide moves out, which is the opposite movement to what takes place in the lungs. To sense this, let your awareness spread out to the whole of your body and come into a sense of your arterial blood flowing out from the heart to the whole body. Try following it as it moves into smaller and smaller arteries. Use the image of the river delta to help you come into a sense of blood reaching its destination – at the body's cells – and of the blood moving into the countless estuaries interweaving through all parts of the body. This can lead you into a very different sense of yourself. This is the place where cells feed and where your deeper digestion takes place. Does your body feel satisfied? Does it feel like it's getting enough? Are you reaching all aspects of yourself? Are you inhabiting yourself fully, engaged in the exchange of nutrients, complete in the process of absorption and release? Is there anything you need more of? Does it feel full, soft, alive with vitality or is there a lack of exchange? Are there any areas that feel cut off or absent, ignored? Ask the questions and acknowledge what comes back to you – that way you can address whatever arises in an appropriate manner.

WHAT'S IN BLOOD?

Your blood is pretty much made up of red blood cells in sugary water. Red blood cells account for 99.9 per cent of all blood cells. The other 0.1 per cent are white blood cells, which are to do with our immune response, and platelets for clotting blood. Red blood cells are amazing. Their sole function in life is to transport oxygen from the lungs to the cells of the body. So important is this function that nature has made sure there are, at all times, around 25 trillion of these cells in the blood of an average adult. That's a huge number and accounts for about one third of the number of cells in the entire body! The image below is of the most numerous cell in your body. It's literally a third of who you are. So take a deep look at it as you are essentially looking at a huge aspect of yourself. It should look familiar and its nature you should know very well, because it's what your body is expending most of its energy on.

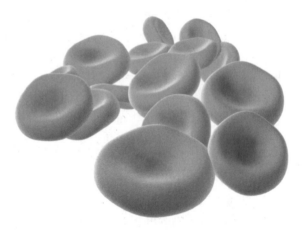

Red blood cells

Nature has designed these cells to absorb large quantities of oxygen. Here's another mind blowing fact: each red blood cell contains 280 million molecules of a special protein called haemoglobin, each of which can absorb up to four molecules of oxygen, meaning that each cell can absorb more than a billion molecules of oxygen! Red blood cells are basically super sponges! That's a vast number of cells carrying an enormous quantity of oxygen around the body, which is just right, because the cells of the body absolutely need it otherwise we grind to a halt.

A red blood cell takes a bit of a knocking in its journey. A round trip through the circulatory system takes about 30 seconds, and the trip is a bit rough too. The cells are banged around by the heart and major arteries, squeezed through capillaries, and after travelling around 700 miles they finally get worn out and start to break down. Therefore, keeping the population of red blood cells constant is vital and requires a lot of effort. Three million new cells per second need to be produced to keep the levels constant and the body furiously produces these in red bone marrow.

You can imagine that due to the landscape red blood cells have to traverse, they have designed themselves in such a manner as to reach optimum efficiency. They are highly flexible and can deform and flow through vessels smaller than themselves without tearing. The red blood cell has a disc shape. Have a good look at the image on the previous page. What does it remind you of? There's something quite pleasing about its shape. It's smooth and lozenge-shaped and looks like a sweet or flying saucer. In order to squeeze through capillaries, red blood cells often stack themselves together like dinner plates. Go on to the internet and search for red blood cells and you will find microscopic photos of them doing just this. You will also see how flexible they are – how they squeeze up to get through tight corners. Notice how red they are too.

BLOOD NATURE/ANIMAL-SELF/WOMB-LIFE

We have a strong connection to the animal kingdom through our blood. Blood connects us to animals by the mere fact that we share the same ingredients and many of the same bodily processes. We once hunted with our own hands, faced the conviction of killing and held the gratitude of the surrendering of another life. There's no denying spilled blood and the loss of life. Today we live in a bloodless society. Animals are still being slaughtered, their blood still being shed, just not by our own hands and so we don't have to face the impact of death. In many religious traditions animals have been slaughtered for the atonement of our sins, a ripe metaphor for the blood inside of us – an offering of life for life – the opportunity to cleanse our souls.

Blood is the medium through which life is carried. When we connect to our blood in an energetic way we connect to something that is primordial, something that is beyond ourselves and at the same time is us. Isn't it interesting that we can share our blood, that the mystery of life is shared by all, connects all and yet, when we bleed it's deeply personal? We simply cannot live without it.

Women are in contact with their blood nature through their monthly cycle and through pregnancy when women share blood with their baby and grow a new blood organ, the placenta. This makes women much more conscious of their blood and their viscera. The visual recognition of blood during the menstrual cycle is a symbol of the loss of an opportunity for a life to be born and through every birth there is blood. It is common knowledge that women living together often find that their menstrual cycles synchronize – a unifying experience that creates a powerful energetic connection to each other and to the cycles of nature.

Likewise, as a foetus we are totally oriented to blood through the umbilicus. How must that have been for us? Think about it: a huge conduit out of our belly into the placenta, blood moving back and forth, feeding off the mother – our lifeline to growth and development. A blood bond, the pulsating and interconnectedness of all life. Blood moving back and forth, the medium shared between two beings, literally. Metaphorically, this relationship transforms into a deep understanding of the reciprocal nature of life that belongs to us all and that we participate in and contribute to.

The very nature of blood is profound in itself; however, blood also brings a certain awareness with it that will be intimate and personal. Bringing your awareness to your own blood flow and being open to what it means to you may lead you into a deeper awareness of yourself that may well be surprising and unexpected. Blood may seem obvious, but its wisdoms are astounding.

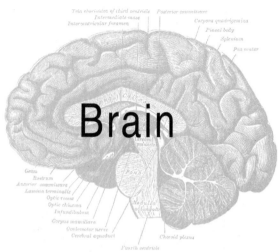

Chapter 7

Brain

HUMANS HAVE BIG BRAINS

Being human we take great pride in how 'big' our brains are and tend to look down on other species with smaller brains. (Animals probably equally think we look ridiculous with our oversized brains.) Actually there's really not that much difference. The basic underlying functions and activities of the brain that occur on a daily basis are the same across all species with a nervous system. Most of what brains do, no matter their size or shape, is fundamentally similar – to coordinate and orchestrate body movement and senses.

In our early embryological development we are simply a fluid-filled tube that will eventually become part of our central nervous system. This is a common link with other forms of life including many invertebrates that have this tube-like nervous system, but particularly the 'phylum cordata' which includes fish, birds, reptiles, amphibians and mammals. The difference, that will eventually separate us, occurs in what happens around this early fluid-filled tube as things develop. In humans, and so-called higher vertebrates, the brain becomes complex, growing in powerful and mysterious ways to become large and

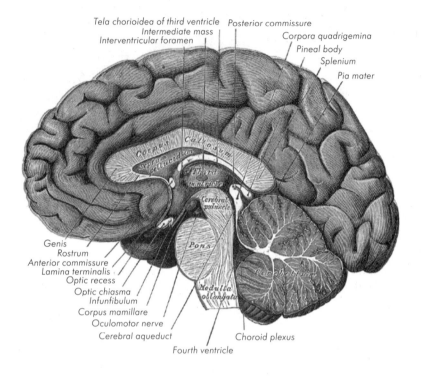

Tela chorioidea of third ventricle
Intermediate mass
Interventricular foramen
Posterior commissure
Corpora quadrigemina
Pineal body
Splenium
Pia mater
Genis
Rostrum
Anterior commissure
Lamina terminalis
Optic recess
Optic chiasma
Infunfibulum
Corpus mamillare
Oculomotor nerve
Cerebral aqueduct
Pons
Medulla oblongata
Cerebellum
Choroid plexus
Fourth ventricle

The brain

globe-like. Yet, despite all this growth, at the core of the brain, the original fluid-filled tube is still to be found, transformed, but remaining a connected waterway.

Interestingly, the one structure we all have in common is right at the core of us. Our development proceeds outward from this fluid space. Our brain has grown on top and around the fluid-filled tube, with the spinal cord growing out concentrically from it, followed by our bones, muscles and organs. We have grown out from an original fluid reservoir. Think about that for a while, as it's a powerful thing to understand. *Our inner nature is fluid and tubular and connects us to most other life forms on this planet.* In many ways there's a wonderful simplicity here, which is a relief as so much of the rest of the body is so highly complex and difficult to understand, especially the brain. It's helpful to remember that at the core of us is this simple fluid tube that is the foundation for our super-complex brain. It's a wonderful combination and, hence, both of these states/realities are within our nature. Perhaps if we paid more attention to the fluids, we'd get some relief from the relentless processing of the brain, with all its constant thinking, reacting and integrating of information as well as responding. All those millions of electrical surges per second can find some relief in the fluids within and around the brain. It's like the fluids need to cool the brain down as all that electrical firing produces a lot of heat. Here's the yin and yang of the brain. Nature has provided us with our very own escape route from the constant activity of our brains. When you do the exercises below you may notice that, as you shift into the fluids, the brain stills and thoughts slow down – a useful tool to survive the 21st century.

BUT THERE ARE HOLES IN IT

It's extraordinary that at the very centre of our nervous system there are big spaces with no brain in them! Large chambers within the brain: two big sausage-shaped ones at the centre of each hemisphere, a doughnut-shaped one deep in the centre of the brain and a smaller diamond-shaped one in the brain stem. They are called ventricles. The centre of the spinal cord is also hollow. A thin tube called the central canal rises into the head to join up with these chambers in the brain. That's pretty wild. Take a look at the image below. This is what's left of the original fluid-filled tube of the embryo. Due to the brain's massive growth, the compression of space has changed much of the original shape of this tube. Despite this you can

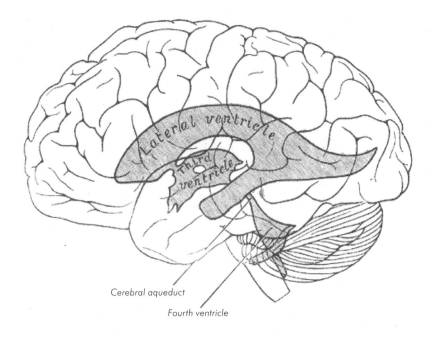

Cerebral aqueduct

Fourth ventricle

see that the big spaces are still attached by small connecting waterways, called aqueducts, which keeps the continuity of all the fluid cavities.

AND IT FLOATS IN A SEA

We live on a fluid-filled planet. All life on this planet mirrors the world it lives on. It's a sea planet, so, you could say, we are sea creatures even though we live on land. The ventricle spaces are like our inner seas, held deep within the centre of our bodies, that have been with us since our formative days. The fluid is salty, our brine, and the brain floats in it.

For years I thought I was nerve, muscle, bone and guts. Now I realize I am also brine. Most of the brine is found in the brain and spinal cord, but you can find it everywhere in the body, in cells and between cells. We are suspended in brine.

This fluid, in and around the brain, is called cerebrospinal fluid. It's a clear, colourless fluid and its composition is similar to blood plasma. It's actually derived from blood through special structures located in each of the ventricles that are essentially blood filtration systems, producing a one-way secretion of fluid from the blood into the ventricles. In effect, it's filtered blood and is controlled for its exact composition. There's not a huge amount of it (about 150 ml), but there's a strong flow (about four times this is produced daily) through the ventricles. Its composition is similar to amniotic fluid that bathes us in the uterus as we grow. The body really likes this kind of fluid. We are pickled in it for the first nine months of life and the central nervous system is always pickled in it. It needs to be pickled in it to function. Picture this: the brain and spinal cord (really these two structures are not separate, but are part of one brain) enclosed in a special bag that is tough and that keeps in the fluid. It maintains a controlled environment. It means the brain can have exactly what it wants: it can float in brine – not unlike a jellyfish. It's like the brain has created an internal sea to keep its aquatic nature intact. The rest of the body is also soaked in brine, but the brain is special as it needs to be reminded of its original nature all the time. Fluids create an optimum environment for growth and development and it is remarkable that the deepest mechanism in our body should hold on to its original structure and maintain a fluid environment.

Exercise: Brain like a jellyfish

How to feel your brain... Start by feeling something different in you that's like no other part of you. For instance, it's not muscle as it doesn't contract, it's not bone as it's not dense in that way, and it's not like the organs of the body either (i.e. the heart, lungs or liver). It's something entirely different. Find a quiet place and place your hands over the top of your head by resting your elbows on your thighs. Relax and stay with the feelings in your hands. At first it might feel hard, but as you stay there for a while you will feel it start to soften and then eventually it will all start to feel more like fluid than bone. This means you are now feeling beneath the bone. The movements can be quite amazing and unexpected, but definitely very fluid-like. The head is filled entirely by the brain so you should easily be able to feel it moving in its fluid space. There's a quality to its substance – see if you can describe it to yourself. The brain is also highly active and you may well feel its electrical nature. You may also be able to get a sense of the brain's extent (i.e. the whole mass of it). See if you can be open to this. When you get a sense of this, you may be able to feel the spinal cord attached below and this is when you may feel like your hands are on a jellyfish bobbing around and buoyed up by the sea. What's your sense? If nothing comes to you, keep returning to the exercise a few times. It's often a matter of becoming familiar with new sensations.

Exercise: Voyage of the tadpole

Sit comfortably and become still. Let your awareness take in your head and spine. At the back of your head and brain, just beneath the surface, is a reservoir of cerebrospinal fluid called the cisterna magna (big cistern). Imagine that you are a tadpole swimming around in this cistern. Use the picture of the brain as your map. Hold the image of the tadpole gently, as you are using it to explore deep and sensitive places in the core of your brain. How does it feel in there? Try swimming around the cistern at the back of your head. You can also swim around the outside of the brain as the brain is floating in fluid. You can swim all the way down to the bottom of the brain and down the length of the spinal cord. As you swim down towards the bottom of the ribs, the space widens and becomes another cistern or waterbed. Great word that, waterbed. They each have their own qualities as different things go on there. Now swim up the central canal of the spinal cord to the fourth ventricle. Spend time swimming around the fourth ventricle, then swim up the aqueduct to the third ventricle. Again, spend time exploring the third ventricle before swimming up into each lateral ventricle. Swim the length of each ventricle before coming back down to the fourth ventricle and exiting back to the cisterna magna. Wow. What a tour! How was the experience of each ventricle?

ON THE BEACH

The next time you are lying on a beach, notice what part of your body is most affected by the sea. If you are not near a beach then imagine lying on a beach. Listen to the sounds of the waves, smell the sea air, notice the horizon. Your body will be strongly affected by this, so try to notice the detail of your body's response – which parts of you are particularly affected? You should find your heart rate decreases and your mind and body relax, but if you pay attention to any deeper feelings that arise, you might find a strong connection to your ventricles – fluid resonating with fluid. Sit a while and observe your response. I wonder if, at a deeper intrinsic level, this is why so many people like being at the sea – not really for the tan!

A BRIEF HISTORY OF THE BRAIN

For hundreds of years the Chinese considered the brain to be a sub-structure of the kidneys. The ancient Greeks thought it was a bladder. The Egyptians thought the heart was the more important organ and paid little attention to the brain. Aristotle suggested that the brain's function was a cooling system for the heart. Interestingly a couple of early Greek physicians decided that the ventricles were the places of intelligence in the brain. Not many people seem to have given the brain much importance, and only relatively recently has the brain been recognized as a remarkable organ in itself. The dominance of the heart has eclipsed the brain for thousands of years and so it's a new phenomenon to have a culture that is brain-centric and maybe that represents the shift in mindset of the modern age. The heart was considered the seat of the soul and the centre of thought and feeling and much of this has shifted to the brain. The last vestige of the heart's dominance is that it's still considered the centre of feelings.

In the 18th century Descartes suggested that the brain was merely an instrument of the mind, which was something non-corporeal. This highlights a debate that has gone on for centuries about whether the brain is the mind or not. This debate continues today with current research revealing that the brain is not just a complex collection of interconnecting wires, but also a hormonal soup. Millions of electrical impulses take place every second as well as the simultaneous production of special molecules that have wide ranging and powerful effects on the brain, affecting our emotional and psychological states. Therefore, the brain is not only an electrical phenomenon, but also a chemical one. Some researchers have gone even further to suggest that some of these special chemicals may actually be the material component of thoughts and emotions.

And what about the body? In many ways the body has been constructed as a housing for the brain and spinal cord. It allows the brain to venture out and see the world and to offer protection. So we are walking, talking brains. The body prioritizes the brain and will try to keep it alive at all costs. The body will cut blood supply off to everything else before it will stop supplying blood to the brain.

THE BRAIN'S IN A BAG

Everything has a skin – plants, animals, planets, cells, atoms and humans. It's part of nature that there's an interior and an exterior to life and skin serves as the medium in between. In humans, we have the skin we all know and talk about and spend so much time looking at and taking care of, which is obviously the one covering our body, but that's just one of many skins. There are so many more skins within your body that you can't see. Each bone and muscle has a skin, nerves and blood vessels too, and of course all the organs of the body. The brain also has its own skin; in fact, so precious and important is the brain, that it has three of them! These are called the meninges (membranes) and they come in different sizes.

The outermost layer is a really thick membrane that connects to the cranial bones and forms a strong protection for the brain. It wraps around the whole of the brain and the spinal cord like a balloon with a tail. However, the balloon in the head has another balloon just inside it. The inner one has a curious structure that looks like an internal Mohican haircut. It makes you wonder how intuitive the Mohicans were with their bodies. This inner membrane has projections deep into the brain both vertically and horizontally. It descends several inches into the brain. The Mohican part of it, which runs from front to back, projects into the space between the hemispheres

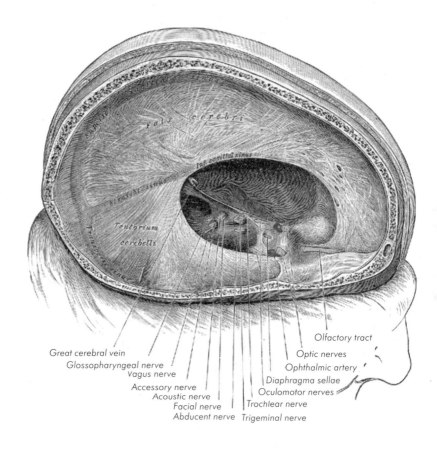

Great cerebral vein
Glossopharyngeal nerve
Vagus nerve
Accessory nerve
Acoustic nerve
Facial nerve
Abducent nerve

Olfactory tract
Optic nerves
Ophthalmic artery
Diaphragma sellae
Oculomotor nerves
Trochlear nerve
Trigeminal nerve

of the brain, and the horizontal one divides the lower brain from the upper brain. These structures keep the brain in place and act like a cross-hatched endoskeleton for support. They are slightly elastic too and can, therefore, absorb any shock from impact, especially since they are directly in contact with the bones of the head. The Mohican-shaped or vertical membrane is called the falx, which is Latin for sickle, and that's exactly the shape it is. The horizontal membrane is called the tent, as it's tent-shaped when you look at it from the back of the head. The other important function of these structures is to carry blood returning back to the heart from the brain. They contain special vessels that allow blood to flow from the front of the head to the back, before moving down and entering the jugular veins and exiting the cranium.

The next layer of skin or membrane is called the arachnoid, because it's got spider's legs on its underside. This is important because it contains the cerebrospinal fluid that moves in the space between it and the deepest layer of all, which has a quality more like cling film, as it hugs to every fold and undulation of the brain's surface.

The outer membrane is called the dura mater and the inner membrane is called the pia mater, which mean 'tough mother' and 'soft mother' respectively. It's an inspiring thought that these skins are mothers that care for the brain and bring qualities of toughness as well as softness.

The spine has all three of these layers too; however, the outermost layer attaches only at the top of the spine and again at the bottom of the sacrum, so that it's like an unattached tube or sleeve that contains the spinal cord and allows your spine and cord to move unhindered.

Essentially, this membrane system (especially the big, tough outermost layer) is the most amazing information system held deep in the core of us. It projects into the head and attaches to the cranial bones, runs the length of the spinal canal and connects with the sacrum, creating a connective tissue core as well as feeding the central nervous system with blood and fluid circulation. It connects up the whole axis of the body, making it possible to create an integrity of communication through these vital membranous structures, offering the brain a direct connection to the pelvis.

When this membrane system is healthy, there's a wonderful fluid tension running throughout the length and volume of it. However, there can be dehydration and strain patterns in the membranes that create torsions/tensions and therefore restrict movement, not just in that particular area, but due to its composite nature, throughout the whole system. This means you can get headaches from an injury to your coccyx or, alternatively, your lower back becomes stiff because you get headaches. Now you can understand the benefit of knowing your membranes more intimately and here's how to do so.

Exercise: Balloons

Put your hands on your head and imagine you are holding a balloon. This will help you become sensitive to the brain's membranes, which are all shaped like this. What you are feeling for is a sense of continuity, as each membrane is one continuous structure. It can feel like the palms of your hands are touching the surface of a balloon. The thickest, most obvious balloon is just under the bones. As the head softens under your touch you will get fluidic feelings, and then the bones will feel like they dissolve, and this is when you might feel something other than bones and fluids. You may suddenly become aware of the whole head rather than what's just under each hand. You may also get a sense of the whole head and spine, because the membrane covering them is one unit – from head to tail. Use your mental image of the balloon and the anatomical image on page 124 to help you relate to your meninges (membranes). How do they feel? They have a distinctive quality of feeling and particular tension to them. When healthy, they can feel slippery and there's a sense of glide within the structures around them. You may discover areas that aren't like this too. The purpose of these exercises is to sit and listen for a while. Repeat the exercises as often as possible, as more and more detail will come to you.

THE BRAIN IS A MUSHROOM

In many ways the brain is shaped like a mushroom. There's a long stem and the mushroom cap has grown so much that it's folded down over the top part of the stem. The deeper you go into the brain the older it gets. The newer brain is what you see mostly when you look at it from the outside: the undulating folds all puckered up that look strangely like the intestines. This is the aspect of the brain that differentiates us from most other vertebrates, by the mere size of it. It got so big that it had to double back on itself and forced the cranium to get proportionately bigger in order to accommodate it. It's the reason why we spend so much time in the uterus during pregnancy, allowing this part of the brain (the cerebrum) to grow mightily and why our heads only just manage to get out of the birth canal. In relation to our size, other animals just don't have anywhere near the same prenatal time and don't have to face the narrow exit.

Brain growth begins early and advances quickly during the prenatal months. Brain development commences within the first month after conception, when the brain and spinal cord begin to take shape within the embryo. By the sixth prenatal month, nearly all of the billions of neurons (nerve cells) that populate the mature brain have been created, with new neurons generated at an average rate of more than 250,000 per minute. This is an explosion of growth that will never happen again in the body. The body's mission, at this time, is to cram as many nerve cells into the head as possible. Not only does the cerebrum undergo this buckling to create more space, but the whole brain and spinal cord create flexures, or curvings, of the neural tube to get even more neurons in – the amazing folding brain! If laid out flat the cerebrum is actually 25 square feet, which is pretty much the surface area of your skin! An amazing and curious fact, especially as the brain and the skin are formed from the same original embryonic germ cells.

The rest of the brain is not that dissimilar to other animals. Underneath the cerebrum is the hindbrain. The hindbrain or cerebellum is often an ignored aspect of the brain, especially when compared to the cerebrum, which seems to attract all the attention. However, it's a remarkable aspect of the brain that acts more like a computer than any other area, with millions of fibres entering into it from across the brain, bringing sensory information indicating the position of the body in space as well as monitoring internal sensory information to identify the position of muscles and joints.

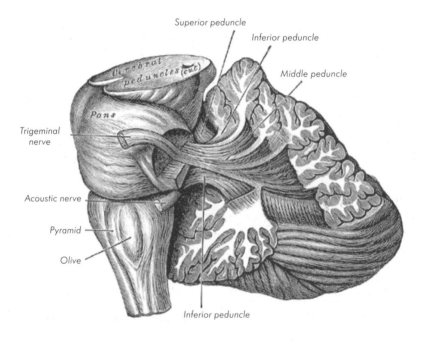

The cerebellum

Structurally the cerebellum has two hemispheres, just like the cerebrum, and protrudes out of the back of the brain stem. Its amazing internal structures are quite beautiful and are called the tree of life.

It plays an important role in the integration of sensory perception and motor output. Many nerve fibres link the cerebellum with the part of the cerebrum that controls movements – which sends information to the muscles causing them to move – and it also links to fibres in the spine that provide feedback on the position of the body in space (proprioception). The cerebellum integrates all of this, using constant feedback on body position to fine-tune motor movements along with equilibrium and posture. It's often called the automatic pilot.

The rest of the brain is composed of the brain stem that ends in a bulb-like structure in the middle of the brain. The middle bit is like the meeting place between the stem and the head of the mushroom, the cerebrum. This middle bit is important (where isn't in the brain!) as there are some key functions that occur here. Right at the centre of it is the third ventricle, which surrounds the thalamus, the name for the top of the stem, which interestingly looks a lot like the head of a penis.

The thalamus is the relay station of the brain. It distributes sensory information that comes in from all over the body to different regions of the brain. The thalamus helps as a dampener of sensory information into the cerebrum, so that the conscious and voluntary parts of the brain don't get overloaded. The other important parts of this area are the hypothalamus and the limbic system, both of which are strongly related to emotional states of being and to production of hormones (to be considered in Chapter 9).

The brain stem is referred to as the reptilian brain. It looks after so-called basic body functions, all of which are unconscious and involuntary processes essential to life, namely those for survival (breathing, digestion, heart rate, blood pressure) and for arousal (being awake and alert). Not to mention the main highway for nerve impulses passing to and from the brain along with special nerve centres that control much of the face and mouth. A really lively place, so no wonder we get neck ache!

Exercise: Feel your brain

Place the palm of each hand on the top of your head so that each of your hands covers half of the top of your cranium. You can rest your elbows on your knees. Feel the different parts of the brain. Under each of your hands is a left and right hemisphere of the brain. See if you can come into a sense of the jellyfish, and when you feel you have a sense of that, notice if there's a sense of two separate structures at the top of it. These are the hemispheres and each one has different functions so they're likely to feel different and might even have different levels of electrical activity occurring. Are there any parts of the hemispheres you are drawn to? Any hot spots? If you stay with it for a while, you might notice the falx between the two hemispheres, which might then lead you to get a deeper sense down into the space between the hemispheres (given the wonderful name of the central fissure) connecting to the bridge that brings them together, called the corpus callosum. This is a busy place as there is a vast amount of inter-relating happening here between the hemispheres. There are 200 million nerve fibres carrying an estimated 4 billion impulses per second. With that kind of communication occurring you can't fail to feel it.

Now move your hands so that the fingers and palms cover the back of your head and upper neck. Right under your hands is the cerebellum. Halfway down the back of the head is a knobbly bit called the inion (which is thankfully short for 'external occipital protruberance'). It's pretty pronounced so you should be able to feel it. This is at the level of the horizontal membrane called the tent. It's the division between the upper and lower brains and you might be able to get a sense of this. It definitely feels different below this line as what you're feeling is the cerebellum or hind-brain. It also has two hemispheres divided by the falx, just like the cerebrum above it. Stay with the cerebellum for a while and notice how it makes you feel. Perhaps you get a sense of the mass of it projecting out from the brain stem and this might lead you to feel the brain stem itself. It can feel like a long rod-like structure rising up from the spinal cord into the centre of the brain. Don't worry if this isn't something that comes to you immediately, as it can take a while to sense the different structures and their particular activity. With practice, you will easily be able to sense all of this. Keep at it.

BE LIKE THE SEA

Think about how fluid-like you are in your life, in your job, in your relationships, in how you think, how you express your emotions, in how your body moves and functions. Remember, at the very centre of you is fluid. This is a fact, not a fanciful idea. By starting to relate to this element in a conscious way you are allowing your innermost nature to manifest itself. Your natural state is hidden deep within you. If you are in relationship to these fluids it leads you to suppleness of body and mind. How is a mind that is fluid-like? The brain, your thinking organ, is fluid. How can thoughts become fixed in an environment that is essentially fluid? That's the mystery. We so easily get caught up in patterns of behaviour and habituated responses to life and become set in our ways. To break out of your habits, try:

- connecting to the big ventricles in the cerebral hemi-spheres and notice how it improves how you think and process information

- connecting to the third ventricle in the centre of the brain and notice how it improves how you emote and relate to others

- connecting to the fourth ventricle in the brain stem and notice how it improves your basic life functions.

Homeostasis means to have a tendency to create balance or equilibrium. At the core of us we have an intelligent system that functions specifically to maintain and nurture a balanced brain and body. Therefore, making connections to these underlying fluid reservoirs in your brain will bring your mind, emotions and body into a balanced state and allow your potential to unfold in your life. Things will start to flow for you. You will see that there is a rhythm to life and events. Imagine, too, how much easier relationships will become when there's an ability to move together in fluid.

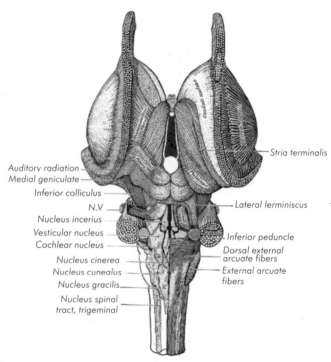

Auditory radiation
Medial geniculate
Inferior colliculus
N.V
Nucleus incerius
Vesticular nucleus
Cochlear nucleus
Nucleus cinerea
Nucleus cunealus
Nucleus gracilis
Nucleus spinal tract, trigeminal

Stria terminalis
Lateral lerminiscus
Inferior peduncle
Dorsal external arcuate fibers
External arcuate fibers

The brain stem

THE SOUND OF THE BRAIN

Finally, listen to your brain. Find a really quiet room in your house and sit still. When you sit still your breathing and heart rate will slow down and they will become less obvious in the body. These are big movements that affect the whole body, but when you become still and relaxed they both slow down and your mind can filter out their effects. As you listen for longer, is there any other movement that's taking place or sound that you can hear? There's no sound in the room or outside, your body is settled and yet, there is a sound. Can you hear it? If you listen you can hear the sound of millions of brain cells firing every second. It's a high-pitched sound that never stops. Your nervous system never rests. What is the sound? Try listening to it for a while and try to name the sound. It's the sound of your brain.

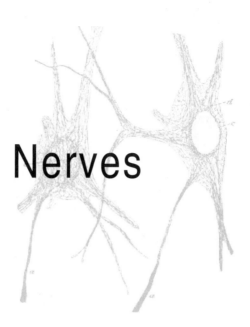

Chapter 8

Nerves

WIRED

Our nervous systems are wired to create a constant flow out from the brain and spinal cord to all parts of the body. This flow is a stream of electrical current that is conducted through the fluid medium of nerve cells called neurons. You know how powerful a conductor of electricity water is. Flow of electricity out generally results in action – movement of muscles, glands or organs. Conversely, there's a constant nervous flow from all parts of the body into the spinal cord and brain, bringing information about the body's state and the environment around it. So there's a constant flow of electrical information coming into the core and reciprocal flow back out to the body to initiate, modify or stop movement or activity. The number of neurons involved in bringing information into the central nervous system is about 10 million, whereas the number involved in the flow out is about 500,000. So you can see how much more electrical current is flowing towards the core rather than outwards, making us humans highly receptive. Our brain is very interested in receiving information and knowing what's going on around it so that it can make decisions and initiate events. Knowledge is everything. However, these figures for nerves look minute in comparison to the number of nerve cells involved in the middle bit, which is about using all that sensory information, making sense of it and then making a decision. Nerve cells involved in this process are called interneurons and are basically neurons talking to neurons, most of which are located in the brain. There are 50 billion interneurons! So to look at it in order of levels of activity: the thing we do least is move; next, by a factor of 20, is sense; and the thing we do by far the most, by a factor of 500,000, is interneuroning. That is, in fact, where all our energy goes! So the next time you feel too tired to move you'll understand why. In terms of the levels of activity in the nervous system, moving takes up such a small percentage of our activity. Actually, less than 0.0001 per cent. You know how much thinking you do – well, consider that that's less than 1 per cent of your interneuron activity. Just imagine the brain energy required to drive its processing activities, which require

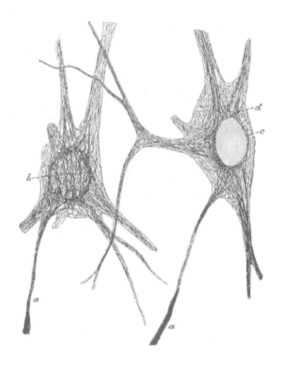

100 times more energy than is required for thinking. Quite a fact to wrap your head around! Our conscious thinking is just a small part of a whole brain that's continuously engaged in unconscious thinking enabling us to make decisions and survive. It's no wonder that half of what you eat goes towards feeding the brain with blood, oxygen and nutrients.

Exercise: Being receptive

Sitting still, bring your awareness to your head and spine. Imagine the bones and membranes dissolve so that you are aware of your brain and spinal cord. Expand this out to include your nerves that run out from the central nervous system to all parts of the body. Be open to being able to get a sense of this. Why not? There's so much electrical activity you can't miss it. Thousands of volts! (Well, thousands of millivolts.) When you have a sense of some of it, sit back even further and try to notice which direction the electrical flow is moving in. It would make a lot of sense if you were drawn to the incoming flow of sensory information. Be open to flow from the periphery to the core of your body. It's an amazing feeling once you tune in to it. There's a real sense of flow from all parts, moving through the body's peripheral nerves in to and up the spinal cord and into the brain. Of course you are feeling something that is happening all the time, but remarkably we miss it at an experiential level. Stay with it and you might well start to relax as you go into receptive mode. This is a big aspect of your nature, remember, much bigger than the aspect of doing/action. You are more wired to being receptive than to being active.

Exercise: Ebb and flow

When you've had enough of experiencing the incoming flow of sensory information, then shift your attention to the other aspect of your nature by noticing the flow of movement out from the spine and head into the rest of your body – electrical flow in the opposite direction. After the last exercise this might take a bit of effort. Stay with it until you are able to relate to this aspect and then notice how different it feels. These nerves go to different structures, but they also have quite a different feel. Try describing them. When you've been with these experiences for a while, broaden your attention out to include the nervous flow in the opposite direction so that you are sensing them together. Here, you might get a sense of the constant ebb and flow of the nervous system: movement in to the core and out to the periphery.

HOW NERVOUS ARE YOU?

The answer, in fact, is what else could we be? There's a vast web of nerves moving through the length and breadth of our bodies emanating from the spinal cord and brain much like the wiring coming out of a central electricity board of a building. What we call nerves are actually bundles of nerve fibres running together just like a copper wire. Open up a copper wire and you'll find many copper fibres within the insulation. Nerves run from the spine into the limbs, trunk and head, and there are two kinds. One kind flows from the periphery to the core, bringing sensory information about how hot or cold we are, what areas are stretched, where things are located in the body, how constricted we may be as well as seeing, smelling, hearing, tasting and balance – what's going on within and around us. The other kind initiates movement within muscles, glands, blood vessels and organs, etc. Nerves travel deep in

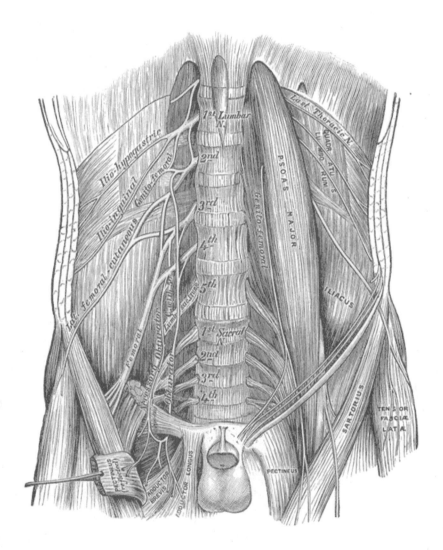

the body, generally between muscles and organs, and through membranes – in a very similar way to blood vessels – so that they are protected from harm. Indeed, you'll find that the two often run together through the length of a limb, in and around the guts and organs.

Clever, that. Insulation is a big thing for nerves as without it the electrical impulse will be distorted and there will be interference just like a TV. The body manufactures special insulation for nerve fibres made out of fat! In a typical nerve, each of the nerve fibres is insulated (there are around 10,000 fibres in a typical nerve), they are bundled together in groups, depending on which way the nerve flows and where they are going to or coming from, and then the whole nerve is wrapped in a special layer. Like nerve skins.

One easy way to understand nerves is to see them as roots and branches of the spine (spinal cord). Here's an image of it. The thing to appreciate is that this is a simplified view showing just the main nerves and not showing all the many branches that stem off from these. Use the image to help you find your nerves in your own body. It will bring a sense of the nervous network that runs throughout your body, how it feels and interweaves through all of the structures and how in many ways you are like a tree.

While you were doing the previous exercise listening to the motor nerves of your body (nerves from the core out to the periphery – activating nerves) did you wonder how you were able to feel these even though you were sitting still and not moving? Obviously these nerves fire up quite dramatically when you move your body, but they also continue to fire even when you don't move. How it works is that a certain number of muscle fibres are continuously wired up to a nerve fibre. The nervous system automatically turns on each nerve fibre so that part of the muscle tightens, tensing the separate muscle fibres in preparation for when the whole muscle is required to contract. There are hundreds of muscles in the body that are constantly being stimulated by the nervous system so that they are in a state of readiness. Each muscle has around 10,000 separate motor units, so there are around 1 million nerve fibres constantly being turned on and off even when the body is static. This is called muscle tone, and without it we would not have the strength to move. We have a built in reflex to tone our muscles, which the brain doesn't really get involved in – it involves only the nerves and the spinal cord.

THE STRANGE CASE OF THE NEURON

Here's a strange thing. As many people know, all cells in your body are replaced at varying rates. The most quickly replaced cells are from the skin, gut and lungs, which makes sense, as they all have surfaces that come in contact with the outside world and get worn out. Other cells are replaced more slowly, like liver or kidney cells or bone cells. There is one cell though that is simply not replaced: the nerve cell or neuron. Basically, the brain stops growing at around the age of five years and then it's downhill from there. As nerve cells die they are not replaced. Scary? Nerve cells, or neurons, do not replicate them-selves. This means that when you die you still have the original neurons you started with. They are the same age as you and are the most permanent part of your body. The rest of your body is continuously replacing itself. Here's a possible answer to the question of who you are: you are neurons. On average we are losing 85,000 neurons a day, which is about one per second. Fortunately, we start with 100 billion neurons. We lose about 31 million per year, which means, on average, at 70 years old we still have plenty of neurons – 98 billion!

The other strange thing about neurons is their shape. They are shaped like a star with a comet's tail coming off it. The tail can be up to three feet in length or just a small part of a millimetre.

NEURONS – STRUCTURE

Neurons are the first cells to be produced in the body. The embryonic growth prioritizes growth of neurons before any other tissue. The nervous system is the first system to be laid down and then the rest of the body forms around it. The growth during this time is awesome at a rate of 250,000 per minute – it's an explosion of growth difficult to imagine. The baby stays in utero to grow neurons.

So precious are neurons that they are held in a special substance called neural glue or neuroglia. There are about 100 billion neurons in the brain and about 1 billion in the spinal cord, and they are surrounded by glial cells which protect, support and provide constant nutrition for them. These cells make up most of the brain as there are around 30 times more glial cells than neurons. They offer a strong barrier to foreign substances such as toxins and microbes. Neurons are surrounded and protected by the three layers of meninges and the huge, bony layer of the cranium and spinal column. That's how vital and important these cells are. Other cells are expendable, but not neurons.

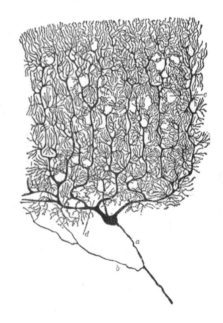

Exercise: Feel your neurons

Hold the back of your head with the palm of a hand. Underneath the bones in the cerebrum are the optic centres in your brain. These receive a flow of electrical impulses from your eyes that is interpreted to give you the sense of sight. Now close both your eyes. Notice the feeling in your hand. Now open both eyes. Feel the difference? Electrical impulses are flowing towards your hand from the action of light on the retina of the eyes. That should feel like a big difference. Now close both eyes and try opening just one eye. Part of the impulses from each eye cross over to the other side of the brain so you should feel part of the occipital lobe light up on either side. It should be more on one side. Try the other eye now. What you are feeling is the combined effect of tens of thousands of neurons.

NERVES HAVE JOINTS

Nerves talk to each other by creating a synapse. A synapse is like a joint. Two nerve ends come together to form a fluid cavity. Electrical impulses release special chemicals at the nerve ending called neurotransmitters that pass across the fluid space and react with the surface of the other nerve creating a response through the whole nerve. Nerves therefore don't quite touch each other, just like joints, plus they have an amazing combination of electrical and chemical actions. The electrical impulse is predictable – it fires or it doesn't. There's a threshold excitation that the nerve needs to reach before it will fire. Bit like an orgasm. The variation comes from what happens at the synapse where the action of chemicals comes into play. Different neurotransmitters produce different effects. There are hundreds of these in the body along with neuromodulators that create a sophisticated response to stimuli. Note that each neuron is in touch with many other neurons. A typical neuron forms 1000–10,000 synapses and there are around 200 trillion synapses in cerebral cortex altogether.

It's difficult to imagine the size of this. Put simply, it means that there is a huge neural web where every neuron is influential and the brain as a whole can react through the synaptic communication system. The amount of connectivity in your brain is beyond anything you can imagine or will probably ever fully use (we utilize such a small part of the potential of the brain). The cascading amount of impulses that can occur through the synapses makes for a challenging visualization.

Once neurons are formed in the embryo, they quickly migrate to the brain region where they will function. Neurons then become differentiated to assume specialized roles, and they form connections (synapses) with other neurons that enable them to communicate and store information. Neurons continue to form synapses with other neurons throughout childhood. At the moment of birth, the large majority of neurons are appropriately located within an immature brain that has begun to appear and function like its mature counterpart. Given the newborn's hunger for novelty, attention to sensory experience and preference for social stimulation, significant changes in the brain's neuronal architecture would be expected after birth. This is precisely what occurs, although the manner in which the brain becomes organized (or wired) in the early years is intriguing. Both before and after birth, an initial 'blooming' of brain connections occurs: neurons create far more synapses with other neurons than will ever be retained in the mature brain. This proliferation of synapses creates great potential for the developing brain, but it also makes the young brain inefficient and noisy with redundant and unnecessary neural connections. Consequently, this proliferation is soon followed by a stage of 'pruning' when little-used synapses are gradually eliminated to reach the number required for the brain to operate efficiently. No wonder children have difficulty regulating their emotional states.

WHITE MATTER, GREY MATTER

We've all heard of white and grey matter, but what exactly are they? The image of the neuron on page 142 will help. The neuron is divided into the body and the fibre. The body has little particles in it called Nissl bodies that give it a grey colour. The fibre is surrounded by fatty tissue called myelin, which gives it its white colour. So white and grey matter are the colours of a neuron. The brain is organized in such a way that there are clusters of nerve bodies and clusters of fibres.

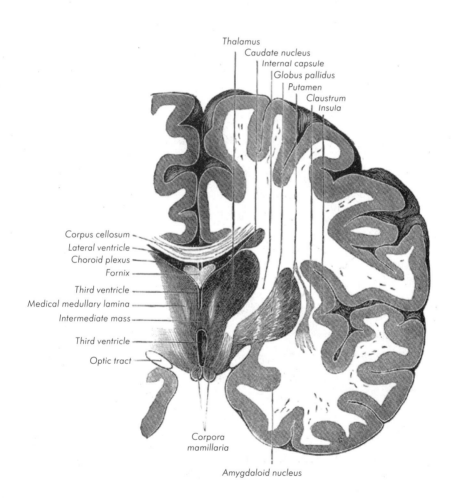

Thalamus
Caudate nucleus
Internal capsule
Globus pallidus
Putamen
Claustrum
Insula

Corpus cellosum
Lateral ventricle
Choroid plexus
Fornix
Third ventricle
Medical medullary lamina
Intermediate mass
Third ventricle
Optic tract

Corpora
mamillaria

Amygdaloid nucleus

Interestingly, most of the cell bodies are on the surface (or cortex) of the brain. So looking at the brain it appears very grey. Looking deeper inside it, though, it looks white.

There are some other collections of grey matter or cell bodies deep inside the cerebrum, in the midbrain and brain stem, but on the whole, most of the inside of the brain is made up of tracts of nerve fibres – a bit like motorways. In fact, 180,000 km of motorway. The grey bit is where the processing (thinking) goes on and the white bit is where the electrical signal is transmitted (i.e. the bit that transmits the thought/information). The spinal cord is different: it's white on the outside and grey on the inside, and if you cut a cross section you'd see that the grey part is shaped like a butterfly and runs the length of the cord.

Exercise: White and grey feelings

Bring your awareness to the surface of your brain for a while, to the grey matter. Then allow your awareness to deepen over an inch or so into the mass of the brain, the white matter. You've gone from sensing the nerve bodies to sensing the nerve tracts. Can you notice any difference? Try to feel it in your body rather than visualize it. Try it again, but this time really spread your awareness across the whole surface of the brain. Stay with that for a while, and then deepen your awareness to be in touch with the whole of the internal mass of the brain. Notice any difference this time? There's much more activity in the grey cortex. This is the core of the neuron, and projecting out from the cell body are hundreds and thousands of branch-like structures, called dendrites, that synapse with hundreds and thousands of other nerves in order to converse. When you deepen into the core of the brain you might have a feeling that you can move across to the other side of the

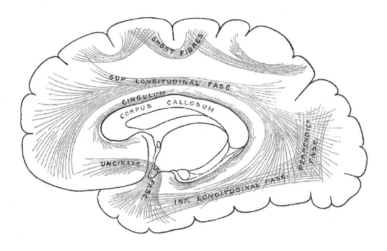

brain, diagonally or in curves, through the brain or down towards the brain stem and spinal cord. This is the experience of the nerve tracts that link the cortex with other parts of the brain and the rest of the body. White is about linear directional movement, grey is about connected processing. Action and comprehension. An inter-relatedness between the two functions. One can't really do without the other and their healthy function is dependent on each system operating fully. What happens if in one level we're able to process information, but struggle to relay it? Somehow getting distracted by the processing and not being fully able to transfer what we've gained. What is then set up in our emotional/chemical responses by the frustrations caused from an internal struggle of brain function.

When you tune in to your own brain matter, what is your experience of these two areas? Do you feel a sense of congruency, as if everything is as it should be, or are you drawn to a particular area that feels compressed? Maybe part of your brain isn't linking up the way it could do? Keep paying attention to what is occurring in your grey matter and then shifting your attention to your white matter. What is that process like for you? Are there parts of your white matter that don't create a sense of connectedness? Is there an interruption to the flow of communication? What does this feel like and what happens to your attention as a result? Interruption creates a communication breakdown and a degree of chaos enters the brain and its processing is less efficient. Spend time meditating on these places within your brain matter and see if you can change your neural architecture. Sounds far-fetched, but why not? There's so much of the brain's potential that we have no notion about and maybe it does have an ability to reprogramme and align itself.

THE SUPERHIGHWAY

White and grey matter continues out of the brain into the brain stem and spinal cord. There's less grey matter in this part of the central nervous system – about 1 billion neurons. Understandably, most of it is fibre tracts bringing and sending impulses back and forth from the brain. We previously mentioned the motorways within the brain, and the spinal cord is like the superhighway for the whole body. Everything has to come in to or go out of the spinal cord.

Here's a really simple view of it. There's horizontal and vertical nerve relationships. The horizontal nerve relationships are to do with the segments of the body. Peripheral nerves branch out horizontally to connect with all the tissues in that segment. You can feel these segments like an electrical wiring system.

Find a friend or family member, sit them in a chair and, using both your hands, make contact with one hand on their spine and the other hand on their body at the same level. Use the circuit map of the body above to feel the circuits. Notice

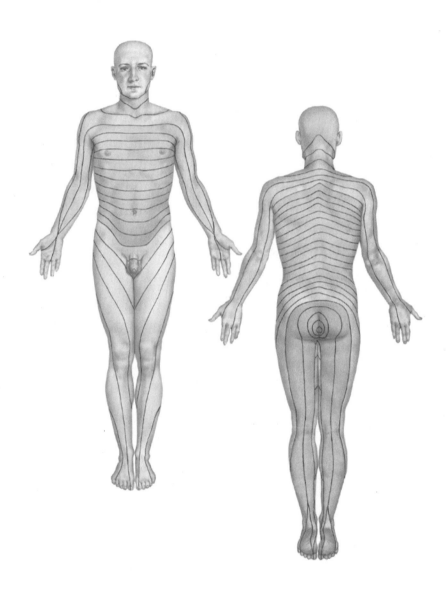

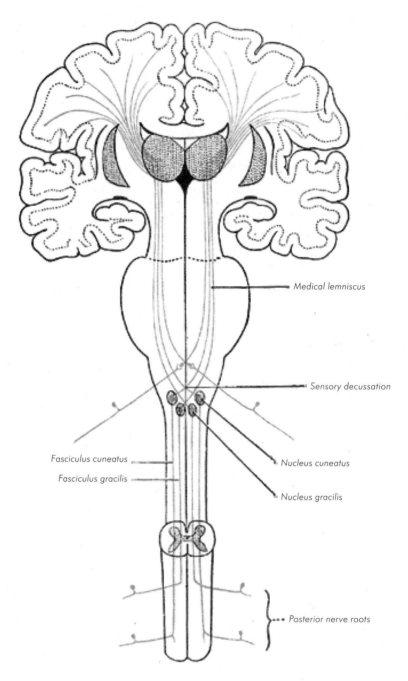

Medical lemniscus

Sensory decussation

Fasciculus cuneatus

Fasciculus gracilis

Nucleus cuneatus

Nucleus gracilis

Posterior nerve roots

The sensory tract

that certain parts of the spine relate to particular areas on the torso or limbs. So if you put one hand around the bottom of their neck, and your other hand on the back of their hand, you should be able to feel a sense of circuit. This can feel like tingling as if you are holding a low voltage electrical wire. Try the same exercise for the chest and ribs. Notice that the further down the body you go the less horizontal the circuits become. The nerve relationships become oblique in the abdomen and pelvis and longitudinal in the legs. So if you put a hand on someone's sacrum and the other hand on the bottom of their feet, you should feel a sense of tingling or connection as if there is a wire between your hands.

Let's follow a typical nerve impulse from your feet to your head. The feet have many special receptors in the skin that create a nerve impulse when stimulated enough. The impulse finds its way to the head through just three cells! The first is from a nerve cell that is as long as the leg (that's its white matter) and has its grey matter located in the spinal cord.

Here there's a synapse with a second nerve cell (in the grey butterfly of the spinal cord) that runs up the full length of the spinal cord in the white matter to the thalamus, at the top of the brain stem, where it synapses with another nerve cell that moves through the interior of the brain to the cortex. The area of the cortex that is responsible for movement and perception of the feet is along about an inch strip of the brain across the crown of your head. Put a hand there and waggle your foot for half a minute. Then hold the foot still and see if you can feel a change. Try it a few times – you might even be able to notice exactly where on the strip the activity takes place.

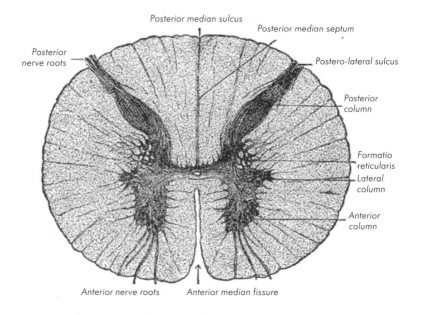

Posterior median sulcus

Posterior median septum

Posterior nerve roots

Postero-lateral sulcus

Posterior column

Formatio reticularis

Lateral column

Anterior column

Anterior nerve roots

Anterior median fissure

Cross-section of spinal cord

MIRRORING

The brain is constantly surprising neuroscientists. New research reveals hitherto unsuspected functions. One of the recent ones is brain mirroring. Cells in the frontal cortex, named mirror neurons, show activity in monkey experiments suggesting they respond empathetically to events in their environment. Neuroscientists believe cells in the frontal cortex are just one kind of cell involved in mirror systems in the brain representing a potential neural mechanism for empathy, whereby we understand others by mirroring their brain activity. That idea is bolstered by new evidence of abnormalities in the mirror systems of people with autism and other disorders that impair their ability to empathize with and understand the behaviour of others. When we observe others' activities, sensations are produced within us that allow us to know what the person is feeling. This can be a whole range of events from pain to enjoyment to much more complex emotional states including other people's intentions. These mirror neurons react to another's brain cell activity. We have become so adept at interpreting someone's body language and facial expressions that we internally reproduce the mental, emotional and kinaesthetic associated states. Listening to your mirror neurons is about trusting your instincts. We are often told to ignore these intuitive responses in our education and parenting, by the media and expectations of society. But if we ignore our body sensations created by our mirroring system, we lose the ability to be highly sensitive and attuned to others and therefore to our environment. I wonder about the mirroring ability of the Aboriginals of Australia or the Kalahari Bushmen, who are adept at reading their environment, or even the mirroring ability of children. It feels like there's something that might have been diminished in our neural pathways. We've got out of the habit of using these pathways so our ability to predict and understand the actions of others becomes inhibited. This leads to a lack of discrimination, reducing your ability to sense danger and protect yourself. We lack the ability to resonate with others and so feel more estranged, less sympathetic and alienated. So bringing about a healthier, more aware relationship with your nerves can create a more discerning and empathetic you.

Considering we're predominantly designed to be receptive to our environment, the decrease in this sensory awareness is catastrophic to the human condition. Is it any wonder that the biggest cause of distress in modern day living is a lack of meaning in individuals' lives? Restoring our capacity to identify, empathize and relate to others will be defined by our ability to connect with our internal senses and trust them.

ONE BRAIN

The spinal cord is the home of our reflexes. Many of our responses do not involve the brain, as they are controlled by the neurons directly in the cord. However, we only make this distinction because the brain and spinal cord have been categorized as separate entities by the medical profession, along with the peripheral nerves. In effect, the nervous system is subdivided into the brain, spinal cord and nerves, but in reality they operate as one system. The nerves are an extension of the spinal cord, which is an extension of the brain. Much like the neuron, with its nerve body, nerve fibre and dendrites – it's all one cell, one unit of function. This is a strong image that doesn't create separation. Your entire sensory perception and activation impulses gather and originate from the whole of the central nervous system. When it functions as a unit, it is at its healthiest, hence, conversely, ill health and disease is often a hallmark of the lack of functionality as a whole. Whilst it is true that the central nervous system is designed in a way that certain areas control associated parts, it is also true that the enormous sharing of information creates a whole brain response. This is the beauty of it and much closer to the reality of how we function healthily. We live in a society that is brilliant at reducing things into compartments and categories, which is powerful in its own way, but there's another aspect of reality that can get lost and that's our holistic response. The response of the organism as a whole. Take this physiological model into your daily life and try living with body intelligence, sensing and intuiting the needs and messages your body is sharing with you all the time. You may find that from this you'll be creating a whole new environment, both inner and outer, true to the perfection of your very own central nervous system.

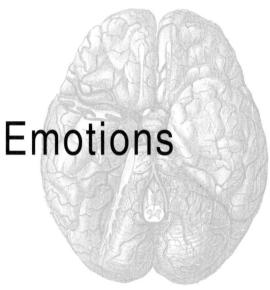

Chapter 9

Emotions

Just how conscious are we? How much of our whole functioning as a human being is in the conscious? That's a question many people from many different fields of knowledge have pondered for centuries. The question from a body point of view can be reasonably well answered through modern biological science. Anatomically we are wired into two main circuits: one which controls muscles and is sensing the external world and muscular movement, and another which controls and monitors the internal world of the organs of the body and has a symbiotic relationship with hormones and hormonal glands. The latter is often called the autonomic or involuntary nervous system because it is literally autonomous and involuntary in that it runs automatically and unconsciously. Thank goodness, as there's so much going on at this level of the body that we would be unimaginably busy and so internally occupied having to make conscious decisions around it. The first system is called the voluntary or muscular-skeletal nervous system and is all about moving your skeleton. As this is such an important function it's given its own wiring in the spinal cord and brain. And a unique headquarters in the brain too. However, when it's described as voluntary that's just part of the explanation. Lots of the sensory information coming to us is filtered out at subconscious levels in the brain. So all that we notice is high-level information. The rest we don't really need to know unless there's an executive decision to be made. The other thing that often happens in this system is decision making by the spinal cord around events that don't need any thought, for instance, reflex reactions like pulling your hand away from a naked flame. The other thing to say is that the majority of communication with muscles via nerves is to do with keeping the muscle fibres in a state of readiness. This is something that is very involuntary. So what's left? High-level sensory information coming from receptors in the skin, muscles and joints, and this is mostly what we are consciously aware of in the body. Overall, this accounts for less than one per cent of all the nervous flux in both systems. So there's so much we do not come into direct relationship with consciously. Add to that a reduction from injuries or traumatic experiences and poor health and the conscious connection to the body's systems can be extremely low. Much can be gained from changing to a more conscious relationship with our body and in particular to the autonomic nervous system. That means getting to know the internal sensory flow from the organs and glands of the body and in doing so becoming more sensitive to your emotional and chemical states.

In this chapter let's explore the details of the autonomic nervous system – the way it functions, the various parts of it, and how to connect to it more fully. Imagine you are walking through the park and from behind the bush in front of you appears a tiger. What's your reaction? Sit with the image and with the sequence of events for half a minute. Can you feel your body response, even though you are only imagining it? What's happening? As I imagine it, I can feel my level of awareness becoming greater. I'm suddenly very present and on alert. My heart is beating faster, muscle tension has increased and my brain has gone into a scanning mode automatically looking for means of escape and trying to calculate the best way of surviving. This is not a time for any other function other than to fight or run. So digestion is closed down, sexual appetite too. You'll not be in a rush to do either of these just for the moment. All blood is being sent to vital organs and skeletal muscles. Adrenaline is being poured into the bloodstream from glandular factories going flat out in the adrenal glands. Phew! That's a big effort. And you can keep it up just for the short term. Back to the tiger, and you've got maybe the best part of 5–10 seconds to make a decision that will enable you to survive. You could run but is there anywhere to run to? Tigers can run really fast over short distances so somewhere safe has got to be close by to make running feasible. Or are you feeling strong? You could attack the tiger. With your bare hands? Or with an object. That might scare it off. Or you could turn into a statue and remain immobile, kind of disappear and the tiger might not notice you, be interested in something else or maybe you get lucky and it's not hungry and just walks on by. All of this process takes place within seconds. Time slows down as your body accelerates internally to produce a massive real-time effect. Let's say after all of that process the tiger stops, looks at you, smells you and turns around and wanders off back round the bush and quickly disappears from sight. What do you do now? Probably collapse on the floor from the shock of it and start twitching and panting as your body recovers from the sudden and huge expenditure of vital resources. It needs time to come back down from an alert mode and to process the sheer relief of having survived. How long this takes depends on how long you've been in this state or how severe the experience. This is called the fight or flight response and is primarily controlled by the sympathetic part of the autonomic nervous system. As we all know from experience, events like these can come in many shapes and sizes. Yet the body will always react as if it's being confronted with a life threatening event even though that might not be the case. As long as we think it's life threatening then we go into an alert state and stimulate the fight or flight response. An extreme version of this is a phobia, but a much more common event is how we interpret situations such as something your boss said to you today or something your partner said that starts an anxiety state within you and takes your body into this process. With animals the survival state is quite simple but with humans the complexity of social interactions has created a spectrum of different responses that can result in a more sophisticated state of being. Included in the spectrum are anxiety, fear and panic, but you can see how these feelings aren't that far away from excitement, exhilaration and elation.

WHERE DO WE FEEL ANXIOUS OR EXCITED?

Everyone knows the answer to this question. We experience these feelings often many times in one day. They are amongst the most experienced emotions and they have specific locations. Remember an event that made you anxious and notice what lights up in your body. It's commonly the top of the chest and the solar plexus and then in the guts. Now think about something that gets you excited and feel what parts of you light up. Actually the same places light up but with a different feeling.

These places are the plexi of the autonomic nervous system and are key places in the body. Butterflies in the stomach are part of this as are stirrings in your gut and sexual feelings. A whole array of feeling tones are created through the activity of these centres. In fact most of the feelings we have emanate from here, whether pleasant or otherwise. Next time you see a horror movie try to follow your body reactions more closely and you will notice how your physiology expresses itself through these centres. This is a mix of nervous flux and chemical activity.

The autonomic nervous system is the emotional nervous system and includes specialized parts of the brain and a separate and unique set of nerves that run through the major organs and glands of the body.

Exercise: Feeling your plexi

Bring your hand to the front of your chest and place it so that the top of your hand is on a level with your collar bones. The cardiac plexus is on the other side of the bony layer of the chest like a necklace on top of the covering of the heart. As long as your heart is beating and you are breathing the cardiac plexus is always active as it innervates the lungs and heart. Notice how active it is. If it feels stimulated, chances are your heart is running too fast and you are breathing too rapidly. They both go hand in hand. As your heart starts to race your breathing has to accelerate to take in more air. This is like panting when you run, but it can carry on even when you are at rest as the nervous system can't come out of that mode. Keep your hand here for a few minutes and you will see that just touching this spot helps wind things down and your heart and lungs slow down.

Now move your hand down to the solar plexus. This is a very powerful nervous centre in the body and coordinates the activity of many of the major organs of the abdomen – liver, kidneys, spleen, pancreas and stomach. The plexus is deep underneath the stomach so it's useful to bring your other hand round to the back of the body mirroring the front hand. Again feel how the nervous energy is here and keep your hands there until it settles down.

Bring your hands down to the area around your navel. This is the enteric plexus for the small intestine. This can either be highly active or underactive so check how it feels in you both before and after you eat. The nervous system here is key to how well you will digest.

Finally move your hand right down to the bottom of your pelvis just above the bony pubic arch. This is the hypogastric plexus deep in the centre of the pelvis. Again you can bring your other hand to the back of the pelvis and feel for the nervous activity here. How does it feel here? This supplies the bladder, rectum and uterus.

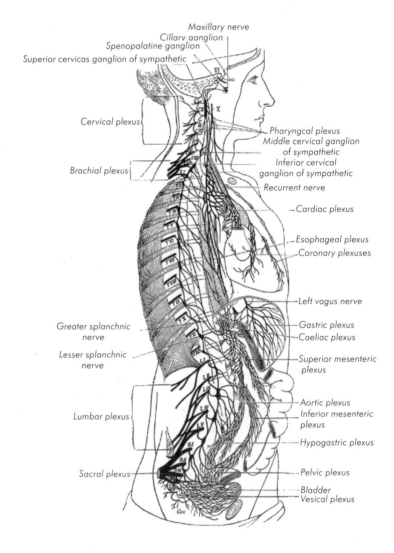

The sympathetic chain

YOUR YIN AND YANG

Your involuntary nervous system is a mixture of opposing forces that create balance. One part of it revs you up and the other part winds you down. The revved feelings are created by the sympathetic nervous system which brings about action. So getting out of bed in the morning, being focused and active, and giving a presentation are all about being yang. Reading this book though is a parasympathetic action, as are having sex, digesting and sleeping. These systems are primal and highly evolved to make us function well. However, in a modern world where there is so much unnatural behaviour, an over-stimulating environment and stressful responses to a pressur-ized world, this part of us takes the brunt of it and is starting to malfunction and break down in many people. It's a testament to the remarkable robustness of the autonomic nervous system that as a species we can sustain this level of imbalance. The prognosis isn't great though. Look around you and you will see the signs of fragmentation: people look fatigued and worn out; sleep problems are massively on the increase along with digestive issues. No one breathes deeply any more and our body systems are breaking down from the inside out, from the organs to the joints, producing poor metabolism and posture.

The neurology of the autonomic nervous system is extensive. It is classically divided into the sympathetic nervous system, concerned with mobilization and excitation, and the parasym-pathetic nervous system, concerned with rest, recuperation and regeneration. There is a dynamic balance between these two systems to maintain homeostasis.

The sympathetic nervous system is a phenomenon of the spine in the chest or the thoracic spine. This is called the sym-pathetic chain and involves two long chains of nerve fibres that run either side of the spinal column close to the front of it.

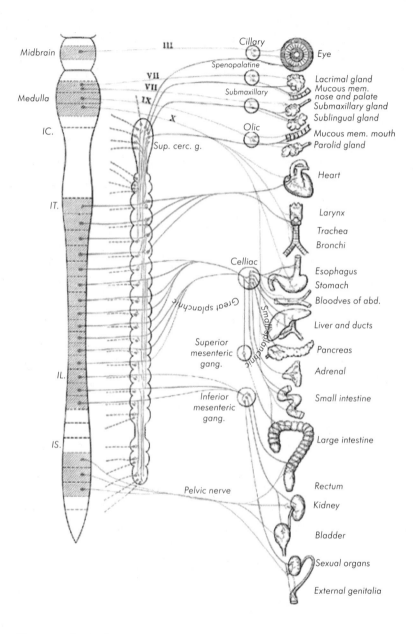

The sympathetic chain

Sympathetic nerves emerge from the spinal column to connect with the chain and then move forward into the cavities of the body to connect with the various plexi described above.

The parasympathetic nervous system is mostly composed of one special cranial nerve called the vagus nerve. Vagus means 'wanderer' and it does just that in the body. It is a huge nerve emerging from the base of the head on either side of the neck and hitching a ride with the jugular veins and carotid arteries into the chest and spreading through the body cavities to connect to all the major organs: heart, lungs, liver, pancreas, stomach, duodenum, small intestine and upper large intestine. That is a massive amount of information carried by one nerve. There are also parasympathetic nerves coming from the bottom of the spine which are also significant as they supply the lower large intestines and the organs of reproduction. So the origins of the parasympathetic nervous system come from the top and bottom of the spine whereas the sympathetic wiring is arranged along the length of the spine in the neck, chest and upper part of the lumbar spine.

If there was peace in the external world and our physical and emotional needs were being met, our homeostatic balance would be wonderful. In a world of constant stress, with no time to rest, we do not have time to resolve difficult experiences that we meet in life, so these become held in the body structure and chemistry creating a congested system that communicates poorly within itself, leading to low energy and depression which are the most common diseases in the world. The lists below describe the symptom picture when these two parts of our nervous response become taxed and irritated. It makes interesting reading.

Signs of sympathetic activation – fight or flight or hyperarousal

- Faster respiration (to get oxygen in).

- Quicker heartbeat and pulse (to supply blood to the large muscles).

- Increased blood pressure.

- Dilated pupils (to take in more light and information).

- Pale skin colour (blood is diverted away from the periphery).

- Increased sweating (there is an expectation of heat being generated in the mobilization response, so sweating can be seen as a pre-emptive response to cool the body down).

- Cold, clammy skin (especially hands, due to less blood in the periphery and increased sweating).

- Decrease in digestive processes (including a dry mouth and contracted sphincters).

- Tingling muscular tension.

- Startle response.

- Increased flexor tension.

- Emotionally this may be experienced as anxiety/panic, terror, aggression and everything happening too quickly and can create overwhelm.

Signs of parasympathetic activation – freeze or dissociation or hypoarousal

- Tonic immobility.

- Numbing.

- Dissociation.

- Analgesia (this may be in the whole body, one side or one limb or a part of one limb).

- Inability to move a limb, dreams of not being able to move (one client called this 'sleep paralysis').

- Inability to perceive the outline of the body (for example, hands or feet feeling too big or too small or too close or far away).

- Inability to feel the skin as a sharply defined edge.

- Sense of floating (this may be the whole body, legs higher than the body or vice versa, or a sense of tilting from one side to the other).

- Sense of disconnection (commonly from below the neck or diaphragm or pelvis or feet).

- Low muscle tone (hypermobility).

- Emotionally this may be experienced as depression, withdrawal, feelings of unreality or not knowing, and lethargy. Dissociation can be a very frightening experience but can also be experienced as a dreamy, floaty, pleasant event – it is a place where you feel no pain.

This is valuable information that could change your life. You will almost certainly have some of these signs. These are increasingly common issues in the world and will seriously undermine your health if you cannot bring them under control. If you feel disconnected or emotionally withdrawn you may well be suffering from parasympathetic shock. If you are constantly anxious and irritable you will be suffering from sympathetic activation. The good thing about the body is that it doesn't lie. If you can listen it will tell exactly what is going on with it.

In fact, it's probably been telling you this all along – you just haven't been listening.

You can help reassert your body's natural intelligence by doing the following exercise.

Exercise: Tuning into the sympathetic and the parasympathetic

Using your awareness, try tuning in to the sympathetic chain and then the visceral nerve network including the collateral ganglia and plexi. Using the pictures of the sympathetic chain (pp.160, 162), see if you can tune in to it. If it is activated it will feel hot and highly charged. Feel the quality and motion within it and the interactions with the organs through the plexi and the visceral spinal tracts up to the higher brain centres. Now tune in to the parasympathetic nervous system from the cranial nerve nuclei in the brain stem (medulla oblongata) and follow it down through the cranial base and the neck into the thoracic chamber and down through the diaphragm into the abdomen through a series of plexi into ganglia at the organs. Notice too the pelvic nerves exiting from the sacrum into the pelvic space and viscera. How does this feel? Is it different to the sympathetic system? Try being attuned to both the sympathetic and parasympathetic systems together and notice how the two interact. If you can stay with an integrated sense of this it will bring about a new balance.

RELAXED PERICARDIUM, HAPPY HEART, LOW BLOOD PRESSURE

There is no doubt neurologically that the body talks to the brain and frequently leads the conversation. The language of the conversation is frequently what we call emotions – the informational chemicals of the neuro-endocrine-immune systems. These

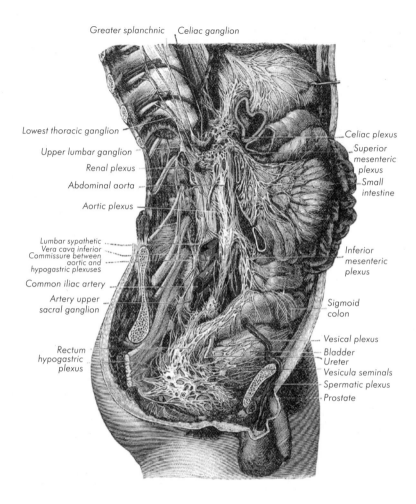

Greater splanchnic | Celiac ganglion

Lowest thoracic ganglion

Upper lumbar ganglion

Renal plexus

Abdominal aorta

Aortic plexus

Lumbar sypathetic
Vera cava inferior
Commissure between
aortic and
hypogastric plexuses

Common iliac artery

Artery upper
sacral ganglion

Rectum
hypogastric
plexus

Celiac plexus

Superior
mesenteric
plexus

Small
intestine

Inferior
mesenteric
plexus

Sigmoid
colon

Vesical plexus

Bladder
Ureter
Vesicula seminals
Spermatic plexus
Prostate

Autonomic nervous system

are mainly produced by the organs and the autonomic nervous system. New science is showing that we can talk of a heart brain and a belly brain. The nervous connections around the heart (thoracic ganglia and its intrinsic nervous system) have their own independent circuits. Similarly the enteric nervous system, coordinating gut activity, has its own independent processing outside the central nervous system (see Chapter 10).

The heart is traditionally associated with emotions and it is true that a lot of your energy and chemical balance comes from the heart. Apart from beating all day and pumping gallons of blood around the body, the heart produces two hormones that reduce high blood pressure and bring your system into a state of emotional regulation. The response to pressure on the chambers of the heart is to stimulate production. However, if there is a long-term stress response in the body and there is tension in the chest that creates a constant pressured environment for the heart, it can lose this vital function. The biggest influence on the heart is its membranous surround, the pericardium. This is a thick protective membrane that maintains a unique chamber for the heart to function in. The pericardium is held in place via strong ligaments that connect it to the diaphragm, the breast-plate (sternum) and the spinal column. It also has connections up to the throat and base of the cranium. So that's a well connected membrane. All these attachments keep it in place and maintain a fixed position so the heart can have room to move within a boundaried space. Stress creates tension. The two go hand in hand. The body response is to make muscles and connective tissues contract and over time this contractile force becomes fixed and migrates to connective tissues that run throughout the muscles and to tendons and ligaments so that joints and membranes become tight as well. Because of the pericardium's many attachments it is very responsive to tensions and strains in the spine, chest and head, and is strongly affected by the breathing mechanism. As it becomes tight it will directly affect the heart, creating a constant pressure that the body starts to normalize around, so that the heart stops responding to it and instead starts to feel like high blood pressure is normal and therefore stops producing its hormones. The body then stays in a high blood pressure state and the heart has to work hard all the time. All of this stems from ongoing stress and mechanical contractions.

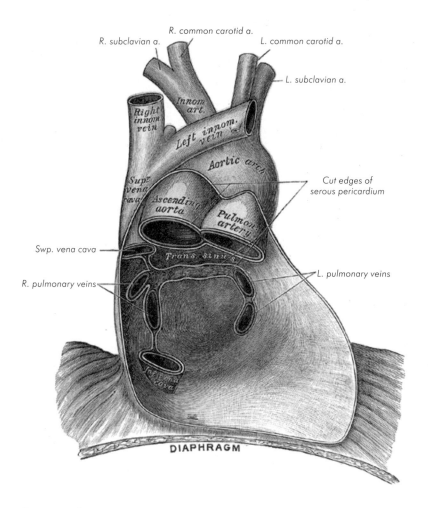

The pericardium

Exercise: Let your pericardium relax

Bring your hand to the centre of your chest. Touch lightly here and let the internal space of the chest come into your touch. This will give you a sense of the organs inside the rib cage and the membranes that surround them. Directly under the centre of the chest is the powerful wrapping of the heart, the pericardium. As you contact here, bring your awareness to your breathing and follow the movement of your diaphragm. Let your breathing deepen and you should start to feel an easing in the centre of the chest under your hand as the pericardium eases up around its attachment to the diaphragm. Now bring the palm of your other hand to the top of the chest, on the spine between the top of the shoulder blades, and hold it there for a while. There is another attachment here that should start to ease up as you continue with the touch. Now move that hand to the front of your throat and notice if there is any tension between your two hands. If there is then stay with the touch and you will notice a natural softening in the front of the throat and in the chest. You can do the same thing by bringing your hand to your jaw. Finally bring your upper hand to the back of your head and notice if there is any tension between the two hands. Stay if there is. Now your chest should feel much more open and at ease and your pericardium will have let go of tensions and your heart will have changed its rhythm. As a result of this your autonomic nervous system will be in a more balanced state and you may feel this change into a more relaxed state.

ADRENAL EXHAUSTION

The body has created a special nerve circuit for instantly mobilizing and moving into the flight or fight mode. This is a coordinated response from the higher brain centres of the hypothalamus and the pituitary and adrenal glands, both via hormonal and direct nervous stimulation. The big problem comes though when there is a long-term stress state in the body and this can quickly lead to adrenal gland exhaustion. Unfortunately, the stress response can become more damaging than the original stress.

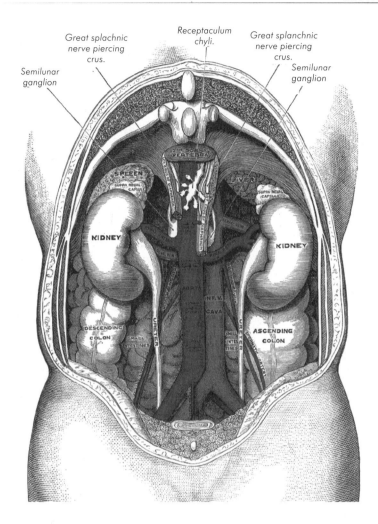

Adrenal glands

Adrenaline is secreted by the adrenal medulla (the deep part of the adrenal gland) within seconds of a stress. Cortisol (commonly called hydrocortisone) is secreted after minutes and for much longer periods. The signal for cortisol release starts in the hypothalamus, goes via blood circulation to the pituitary and then via blood to the adrenal cortex (the outer part of the adrenal gland). Cortisol is a steroid hormone produced in the adrenal cortex. There is very strong evidence linking prolonged cortisol secretion to many diseases, including heart disease, diabetes, poor immune function and growth disorders.

The main hormones of long-term stress are DHEA (dehydroepiandrosterone) and cortisol. Other adrenal hormones, which include adrenaline and noradrenaline, are secreted in short bursts in response to a threatening situation. The body needs balanced levels of DHEA and cortisol to function smoothly on a daily basis, so when there is a shift from normal levels there is a movement away from homeostasis and the body becomes less efficient and less intelligent in its response to its environment.

The short-term stress response is adaptive. There is a 'logic of delay': we shut down everything that is not essential to dealing with immediate danger. All resources are geared to fleeing the tiger. The problems come with continued activation of the stress response. The changes become maladaptive and cause widespread health issues. Reproduction, growth, immune activity and digestion are all switched off when we are running from the tiger. Our heart and lungs and big exercise muscles are working overtime.

Stages of adrenal exhaustion

The first stage, which is called hyperadrenalism, is characterized by abnormally high cortisol levels and subnormal DHEA levels. With the high cortisol levels you may still have energy, perhaps too much, and you may not be sleeping well or restfully. You may be losing muscle mass because cortisol cannibalizes muscle for energy, resulting in weakness. It also causes moon face and weight gain around the trunk, as well as fluid retention and glucose intolerance. Cortisol decreases serotonin levels which may cause depression, and also decreases melatonin levels which adds to poor sleep. It is also immunosuppressive

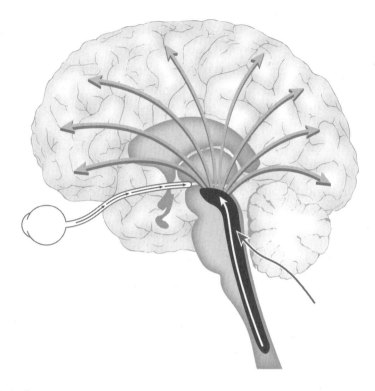

Reticular system

which may result in frequent infections and illness. High corti-sol can cause hot flushes in women. Sugar cravings, confusion and muscle weakness may also occur.

The second stage is where cortisol supplies have finally run low but have not yet run out. For a year or so, cortisol and DHEA will hover in the low–normal range, leaving you feeling tired and stressed, but functional.

The third stage is where cortisol and DHEA levels are low for most of the day, leaving you with low energy levels. Common signs and symptoms of adrenal exhaustion include: inability to tolerate exercise, depression, dark circles under the eyes, lack of mental alertness, headaches, oedema, salt and/ or sugar cravings, feeling tired all the time, feeling mentally and emotionally overstressed, light headedness, heartburn, low blood pressure, recurrent infections and trouble sleeping.

As you can see, if this continued on for some time it would have very serious effects on the body's ability to function normally and would end in illness. Adrenal exhaustion or adrenal fatigue is a 21st century stress syndrome. It has been estimated that 80 per cent of adults suffer some sort of adrenal fatigue, yet it is one of the most underdiagnosed illnesses in Western society and is poorly understood by orthodox health care. Commonly referred to as 'burn out', adrenal fatigue can be caused by: stress (physical, emotional or psychological), lack of sleep, overexertion, poor diet, alcohol, smoking, caffeine, too much sugar, allergies, infections, toxins, excessive copper levels, heavy metal toxicity, fear, marital stress, problems at work, death of a loved one, illness, accidents, negative attitudes, drugs, candida, parasites, etc.

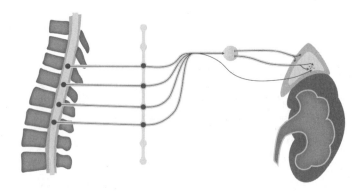

Adrenal circuit

Exercise: Turning off your adrenals

You can really assist your body in shifting out of adrenal burn out by doing some simple things. The first thing to do is to put your hands directly on to your adrenal glands which sit on top of your kidneys. They are not connected functionally but are just neighbours. So if you bring the palm of your hands to the lower ribs at the back of your body, above your waist and close in to the spine, the adrenals will be an inch under your hands. Keep your hands there for a couple of minutes and notice what happens. Touch itself creates a deep physical response that helps to bring about chemical and metabolic balance.

Breathing and heart rate are powerfully affected by adrenaline, so helping your body to slow both of these down will start a feedback mechanism in the body that will help to turn off the flow. Encourage your breathing to slow down and deepen in its movements. Put your hands on the centre of your chest over your heart and listen to the beat. You will notice the heart naturally start to slow down when you do this.

Help stimulate a parasympathetic state by putting one hand on the back of your head and the other on your sacrum at the bottom of your spine. This will help to stimulate the nerve centres associated with the parasympathetic nervous system. Quite quickly you will notice how it activates and starts to balance your whole autonomic nervous system.

Other things to try:

- Think happy thoughts – thoughts and emotions create a physiological state that changes your body chemistry. A flood of new chemicals will suffuse your nervous system and slow down the stress response.

- Eat food you really like – stimulating your limbic system through smell and taste is a very powerful facilitation of the nervous response and will quickly lead to the gut turning back on.

- Wind your brain stem down – see below…

BRAIN STEM LIKE A LIGHT BULB

The brain stem contains nuclei that control the autonomic nervous system. There is a 'magic inch' in the brain stem that controls the heart rate, levels of brain activity, breathing and digestion. The reticular formation strongly connects the brain stem to the limbic system (the emotional brain) and to the cortex of the upper brain. It's a complex neural network in the central core of the brain stem that monitors the state of the body and functions in such processes as arousal, sleep/wake cycles, attention and muscle tone. When the body goes into fight or flight mode it becomes highly activated, bringing the whole brain into a state of hyperarousal.

There is a direct neural signal to the adrenal medulla from the brain stem. Sympathetic nerves connect directly into the adrenal medulla. This causes adrenaline to be released into the bloodstream within fractions of a second in response to a stress. This surge of adrenaline gears the body up for activity – we go into fight or flight mode.

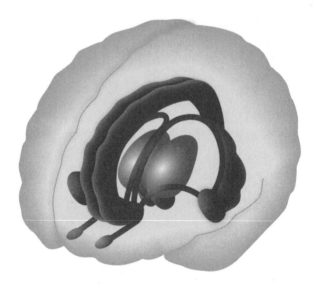

Limbic system

Parasympathetic activity is also mediated through the brain stem. In overwhelming stress, brain stem nuclei, in response to limbic system signals, will trigger the release of endorphins. The endorphins flood the central nervous system and inhibit incoming signals. This is the freeze or dissociation response.

The brain stem can be perceived like the stalk of a cauliflower, below and deep into the hemispheres. It can be perceived as a dense, active core to the brain which connects the fluid ventricles and the lighter, more spongy, diffuse hemispheres to the information superhighway of the spinal cord.

The brain stem is a very powerful portal into working with activation of the whole central nervous system. Activation describes the process where parts of the nervous system become oversensitive and overactive. This is often due to aberrant incoming sensory information (for example, from traumatic events, joints being out of position, organ inflammation, tight connective tissues). The nervous system is not a dry telephone exchange – it is a very fluid place. Neurotransmitters can spread outwards from different neuronal pools of the various nuclei and cause non-optimal firing of surrounding neurons. In this case the nervous system can be said to be activated.

Exercise: How busy is your brain stem?

The brain stem can get very wired up, particularly along a strip of nerve bodies called the reticular formation. So lie down and wrap your fingers together and cup the back of your head with your interlocked hands. Your elbows will be out to the sides of your head. Let your head go heavy into your hands and relax. This will help your brain stem to rev down and that will start a change in the activated state of your body. Your brain stem is bulbous at the top as it comes into the central part of the brain. Imagine that your brain stem is like a light bulb that is turned on. Use the image to slow the activity down by imagining you are turning a dimmer switch to turn the light bulb down until eventually you turn it off. You will notice a strong response as you do this that will result in bringing this part of the brain down to normal levels of activity which will result in the higher portions of the brain following suit. The brain stem activity underpins all of the central nervous system activity and will affect the whole brain.

WHAT HAPPENS WHEN WE FEEL JOY AND FEAR?

The experience of emotion is fundamental to the human condition. Emotion involves the entire nervous system, of course, but there are two parts of the nervous system that are especially significant: the limbic system and the autonomic nervous system. Emotions and feelings, like wrath, fright, passion, love, hate, joy and sadness, are mammalian inventions, originated in the limbic system. This system is also responsible for some aspects of personal identity and for important functions related to memory.

Throughout its evolution, the human brain has acquired three components that progressively appeared and became superimposed, just like in an archaeological site: the oldest is located underneath and to the back, the next one is resting on an intermediate position, and the most recent is situated on top and to the front. They are, respectively:

- *the reptilian brain,* comprising the structures of the brain stem and cerebellum, the oldest basal nuclei, and the olfactory bulbs

- *the mammalian brain,* comprising the structures of the limbic system

- *the new brain*, comprising almost the whole of the hemispheres made up of the new cortex and some subcortical neuronal groups. It corresponds to the brain of the primates and, consequently, the human species.

These three brain layers appear chronologically during the development of the embryo and the foetus, running through the evolution of animal species, from lizards up to homo sapiens. They are three biological computers which, although interconnected, retain their unique types of intelligence, subjectivity, sense of time and space, memory and mobility. So we have three cerebral units in a single brain. The primitive one is responsible for self-preservation. It is there that the mechanisms of aggression and repetitive behaviour are developed, along with the instinctive reactions of the so-called reflex arcs and the commands which allow some involuntary actions and the control of visceral functions (cardiac, pulmonary, intestinal, etc.), indispensable to the preservation of life.

The last decade or so has seen a radical reframing of emotion based on neurobiological research. It has become accepted that it is not possible to make decisions without being able to experience emotion. This is therefore an interactive response between all three brains: the higher brain and the limbic system in connection with the brain stem. Research into trauma has highlighted the unique processing of fear. If we do not feel safe, all the functions of the body are hijacked by the signals initiated from the amygdalae in the limbic system. The amygdalae are two almond-shaped groups of nuclei located deep within the medial temporal lobes of the brain in complex vertebrates, including humans. Shown in research to perform a primary role in the processing and memory of emotional reactions, the amygdalae are considered part of the limbic system and are vital in the process of emotional learning.

We don't feel happy when we are stressed for long periods of time. Chemically it's almost impossible. So the first thing to do is de-stress your body and bring your nervous system into balance. Then the higher centres and the parasympathetic state can start to become more assertive. The higher centre involved in being happy is the limbic system which is a collection of different parts of the brain and spinal cord that operate as a functional unit. This is a mixture of nerve centres and pathways and hormone secreting glands.

Exercise: Smell and your emotional centres – bringing your limbic system into balance

The oldest sense in your body is the sense of smell. Signals from the smell go directly into the limbic system and allow the deep parts of the brain to understand the world outside the body. This all goes on automatically and we often are not aware of how we are responding to other people's odours. Often it manifests as an instinctual feel about someone. So become more aware of your nose and the movement of air in and out of the nasal passages. Follow the air as it moves upwards to the top of the pharynx behind the bridge of the nose. It can feel like you are breathing into your brain, and you nearly are as there is a very thin partition here between the air passages and the internal space of the cranium. There is a thin and delicate bone called the ethmoid between your eyes that has a flat central plate with lots of little holes in it for the olfactory nerves to pass through. These are the nerves that are sensitive to molecules in the air and their stimulation creates nervous signals that move down the length of the nerve and directly into the centres of the limbic system including the hypothalamus, the olfactory bulbs and the amygdalae. If you follow this with your awareness you will be led into this part of the brain and may get a sense of its shape within your head. It has a particular curling shape that is made up of different fibre tracts and nerve nuclei. Let your awareness rest here and you should feel a natural shift to a more balanced state. You may also feel other parts of the nervous system and body responding to this.

WHOLE BODY EMOTIONAL RESPONSE

The body leads the mind as much as the mind leads the body. The body and mind speak and it is a two-way conversation. A large part of this conversation is transmitted via emotions.

Emotions are an embodied phenomenon. The surge of energy you feel when adrenaline is secreted is frequently the emotion of anxiety or excitement. The connectedness and empathy you feel when oxytocin is secreted is frequently labelled joy. The different pieces of music played by the orchestra of cells secreting informational chemicals in our bodies are different emotions. Emotions emerge from the internal environment of the body. They are a particular pattern of secretions and musculo-skeletal tone.

One of the great gifts that emerges from awareness of our bodies is the ability to interact with the process of emotion emerging from the internal environment. A physiological state becomes an emotion which becomes a feeling which can trigger thoughts, reasoning, memories and actions. Understanding this order of information processing leads to many insights about your responses.

There is no hierarchy between mind, emotions and the body. Emotions are not different from or more important than the body. For every mental emotional event there is a correlate in the world of sensation. Actually the sensation comes first – conscious awareness gets in on the act later.

The separations we can make between the body, emotions and thoughts become increasingly uneasy. There is just an organism responding to its environment. We do not exist as an emotional person or a physical person or a thinking person – we exist as a whole unit of function. We respond with the whole of who we are.

Exercise: Whole body emotion

So far we have looked at how the body has specific structures and functions around emotional behaviour and expression. However, are we limited to just these particular parts of the body when we express emotion? Emotions can be so strong that they seem to emanate from all parts of the body as if all the cells of the body are involved. Lots of different parts feel like they hold emotions and these places can be anywhere in the body. As we respond to distressing events around us we respond as a whole unit of function and not just with our particular emotional structures. Commonly we can lock away emotions in joints, muscles and bones, as well as the organs and the nervous system. Sit comfortably in a quiet space and bring your awareness into your whole body. Do this gradually so you begin with awareness of your head and spread out to include the chest and upper limbs and slowly take in your whole torso and legs. Be aware of the volume of your body. Sit with this and you will notice places that feel free and easy and places that feel tight and constricted. One has a feeling of expansiveness and openness and one has a feeling of tension and contraction. If you let your awareness rest into the area of contraction you will come more into relationship with the discomfort of this place, but commonly there will be an emotional content here that is part of the pattern of contraction. As the area becomes too uncomfortable, shift your awareness back to a place of ease and expansiveness for a while before returning back to this place of discomfort. You should find that as you do this there is an easing up of the area and often emotions that are caught up with this pattern start to emerge at the same time as the body starts to reorganize physically in the area. This process is taking place because you are bringing a whole body awareness to this place and that allows a joining up and coming together into a new wholeness. The process is quite natural and automatic, showing that the body and all its different systems desire to operate as one whole body.

WHAT'S SO AMAZING ABOUT THE HYPOTHALAMUS?

This is the magic centimetre at the centre of the brain. It's a collection of nerve nuclei that perform the most diverse array of functions. If there is someone driving the body they would be sat in the hypothalamus as it is the centre of the body. There is nothing like the hypothalamus and its activity and number of functions are inspiring. It is often called the brain of the brain. The overall focus of the hypothalamus is to monitor the body state through blood analysis and information from both the general and special senses. It's an information-gathering machine and based on all of this information it can change the body state through the action of hormones and the autonomic nervous system. It has many functions and here are the main ones:

- controls autonomic functions

- emotions

- sexual behaviour

- endocrine functions

- homeostasis of temperature, hunger, thirst, blood pressure

- motor functions

- regulates food and water intake

- regulates sleep wake cycle.

So the hypothalamus is involved in the majority of the body's primary activities, which is not bad for just 1 per cent of the brain's mass. Clearly, if the hypothalamus is healthy then you are healthy, and if it is not then there are very global consequences. Some of the most severe illnesses come from hypothalamic dysfunction. Here's an exercise to make contact with your hypothalamus.

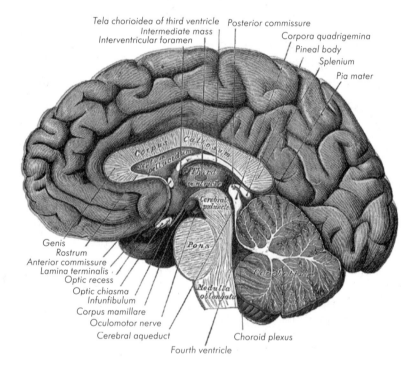

The hypothalamus

Exercise: Finding your hypothalamus

How do you connect with such a small part of the brain that lies so deeply within it? Simple: follow the bloodstream into the brain and one of the first places the blood goes to is the hypothalamus. The hypothalamus is highly active and once you bring your awareness to that area of the brain you can't miss it. Let's start with coming into a sense of your carotid arteries which carry your blood up from the heart to your head. This is a river of blood and if you bring your awareness into your neck it's one of the busiest places there. You should notice three things in the neck: the hollow trachea and the movement of air back and forth, then the spinal cord in the vertebral column behind it and the buzz of the nervous system, and either side of the trachea you will notice a strong flow of blood as it moves up towards the underside of the cranium. Follow this with your attention and you will feel like you are being taken up through the bony layer at the bottom of the head into the inside of the cranium. The carotid arteries emerge at the floor of the cranium and at the bottom of the brain to form a circular arterial structure called the Circle of Willis. This is like a ring main for the whole brain and from here arteries branch off in all directions to move between and into all the lobes of the brain. Right at the centre of this ring sits the pituitary and the hypothalamus is just above it. There are arteries that come directly off this ring to provide blood to both these structures and there are rich capillary beds around both of them. See if you can get a sense of a ring of blood at the bottom of your brain and you will be drawn into the centre of this into a place of high activity. As these structures are both glands, blood flow here needs to be rich and non-congested to allow monitoring of blood constituents and release of hormones into the bloodstream. Let your attention reside here for a few minutes so you can start to get a sense of the natural quality of this place. You will notice just by bringing your presence here there is a strong response across the whole body.

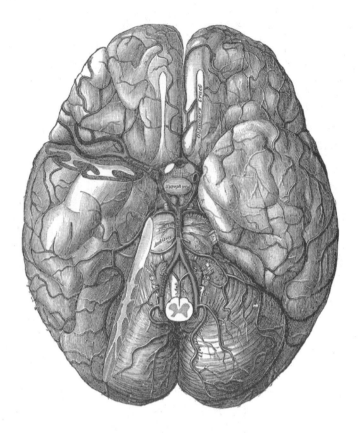

The Circle of Willis

EMOTIONS, STRESS AND YOUR IMMUNE SYSTEM

Over the past 30 years, research has led to a new understanding of the body as a nervous wired system alongside a complex cellular communication, all surrounded by a hormonal soup. Stress is thought to affect your immune function through emotional and behavioural manifestations such as anxiety, fear, tension, anger and sadness, and physiological changes such as heart rate, blood pressure and sweating. These changes are beneficial if they are of limited duration, but when stress is chronic, the system is unable to maintain equilibrium. The HPA (hypothalamic-pituitary-adrenal) axis activity and the inflammatory response are intrinsically intertwined. Put simply, if you are unable to resolve emotional stress you will inevitably be reduced in your ability to deal with infection. This phenomenon may well have started in the emotional centres of the brain but it can quite quickly result in your bone marrow production of white blood cells decreasing.

There are several very important processes to understand in the body's response to its environment. If you breathe badly and eat poor quality food, your immune system will be reduced, making you more prone to infection and disease. Gut irritation produces an irritated nervous system that sends the whole body into a stress response. This in turn means cortisol is being produced that affects the inflammatory response and production of white blood cells. The other consequence is that your metabolism is reduced. Your cells are therefore not receiving enough raw materials to produce sufficient cellular energy to function efficiently, nor are there the right materials to renew existing structures. One of the first things to break down is the functioning of the cell membrane. The membrane becomes less intelligent and starts to lose its ability to maintain a constant internal state, so there is leakage and poor movement across the membrane slowing the whole system down. This is congestion at a cellular level. Cells also start to lose their ability to differentiate key molecules and more critically each other. This is a vital function in the immune response. So toxins, viruses and bacteria are not so readily identified and when they are, the response is sluggish.

Production of white blood cells is a big effort for the body and if there is not enough energy available to drive this, your ability to fight off these intruders is reduced. Some of the first signs of this are an increased sensitivity to substances such as pollen or wheat. Allergies are constantly on the increase in the modern world. Regularly coming down with infections, irritation of the lungs producing chronic lung conditions and irritation of the gut producing irritable bowel syndrome. These are all part of the same phenomenon. All of this can happen very quickly when there are layers of stress.

A similar process takes place when we become emotionally distressed and are unable to resolve it. Quickly many centres in the limbic system become agitated and this turns on the fight or flight mechanism which in turn produces a long-term stress response which leads to gut and breathing issues. When the body is involved in this mechanism it turns off the gut, so that's why food feels like it is just sitting there and your belly becomes swollen. Your breathing shifts into a rapid movement readying you for action but persists even if there is no action. Your heart rate is elevated and there is an increase in blood pressure so that blood moves out from the core to the periphery to enable your muscles to charge up. Obviously there is a similar change in the nervous system. These are all the same signs and symptoms as before but this time they are cascading down from the emotional centres of the brain.

What's the answer to this?

- Recognize what's happening in your body. Notice the signs. Knowing and understanding what is happening to you is transforming.

- Slow down your breathing. Keep reminding your body to do this as it is the fastest way to click off the stress response.

- Eat regularly a well balanced diet. Avoid food your gut reacts to. In time as your system shifts into a more balanced state your gut will become less reactive and more able to tolerate these foods.

- Move your body. This will help to dissipate and discharge the held nervous and chemical energy from pent-up stress.

- Keep in relationship with your body. Bring your awareness to body sensations. Touch your body and come into felt sense, and keep reminding yourself to do this. Do practices that increase this – internal movement sciences, such as Yoga, Tai Chi, Chi Kung, Feldenkrais, that promote body awareness as part of the practice.

- Look at your emotional states. If you are emotionally stable you will be healthy. Balance in your limbic system and autonomic nervous system is best brought about by creating an emotional equilibrium, so avoiding emotional surges and dysregulation will allow your physiology to function smoothly.

- Listen to what your body needs beyond its cravings. Notice what makes you feel good in body and mind. Stay with these things and let go of habits or relationships that don't promote this.

Exercise: Feel your chemistry

Close your eyes. Be with a sense of your whole system. This is the integrated you. Now shift your perception to a sense of individual systems within the whole, such as the nervous system or the gastrointestinal tract. Shift your perception again to the world of individual organs and structures. Notice the kidney, or individual bones.

Shift again to the tissue field. Notice the different kinds of tissues in the body and how they blend together. Shift again to a sense of the cellular level of the body – a sense of extracellular fluid matrix and intracellular fluid and of different kinds of cells.

Shift again to the molecular world within you. This is the level of your body chemistry. Of hormones and neurotransmitters and chemical reactions. What comes to you now? What does it feel like to be attuned to your chemical state?

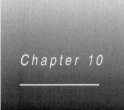
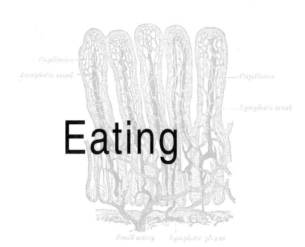

Chapter 10

Capillaries
Lymphatic vessel — — — *Capillaries*
Lymphatic vessel
Small artery *Lymphatic plexus*

Eating

VOYAGE OF A MORSEL

Choose a morsel of food, anything that you like, and follow the voyage it makes as it moves through your gut. Don't eat something too big. It can be a nut, unless you are allergic to nuts, then a grape or a blueberry. Something small and unassuming! Let's do it like a real-time meditation. So don't read this chapter before you have found your morsel. Find a morsel of food first, put it in your mouth and start reading. As you go through the process of digesting and absorbing your morsel, you can digest and absorb the information in this chapter and experience the fantastic process of your digestion.

As you chew the morsel, notice the digestive process starts to take place in your mouth immediately. In fact before it's in your mouth. The smell, sight and touch of it starts off a chain reaction, and before that the thought of it starts it off. Just like Pavlov's dog you start salivating straight away. Enzymes in the saliva start to break its structure down. Keep chewing so you can notice the details of chewing, something you've done billions of times before. Notice too the urgency in your body. Your whole body is gearing up to digest, even though it's just one morsel. The whole digestive tract is being turned on. All

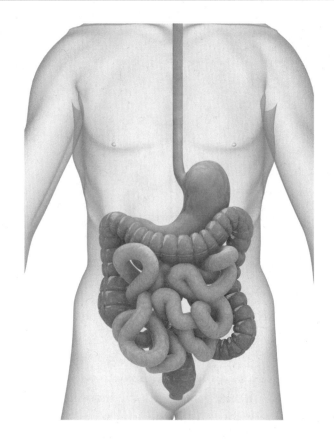

The gastrointestinal tract

the way from the mouth to the stomach, intestines and to the rectum and anal sphincter, it's being stimulated along its whole length. The picture below is the human gut or gastrointestinal tract, GIT for short. The GIT is one whole unit of function. Anatomically it has been given lots of names to describe each section but it was born as a tube and it still is one. So in a healthy GIT when you think of food the whole length of it will get turned on, literally: salivation, mucus secretion, acid production, peristalsis, etc.

The process of digestion is so taken for granted. Breaking down food is a chemical miracle. Billions of reactions are needed to digest the morsel you are eating. That's why your guts are so long – 20 feet in most of us. It takes a while to break food down and it needs lots of surface area, so that once the mouth and stomach have broken things down a bit the small intestine (the next stop on the way down) is where it really happens. This is where we truly feed. Nutrients from the food are absorbed into the body along the length of the small intestine. It's called the small intestine because of its small diameter compared to the large intestine which is much wider.

Let's wind things back a bit to the morsel in the mouth. You can swallow it now and feel what happens. Your oesophagus moves the morsel in a wave down towards the stomach. Normally the oesophagus sits flat in the body except when food passes down it and you can feel this distention as the food moves down through the chest between the aorta and the heart. Acid in the stomach is already being produced so when the food arrives it immediately starts being broken down. If you listen closely and put your hands over your stomach at the solar plexus and slightly left under the ribs, you will feel the stomach doing its characteristic churning which is an interesting mix of side to side movement and front to back movement all caused by three sets of muscles organized in different directions. After a few hours the stomach will break down the food and secrete it into the small intestine and then the pancreas and gall bladder become active and start secreting to break the food down even further. Once in the small intestine, absorption of the food occurs. This is where you will feel constant peristaltic movement taking place and then even stronger constant peristalsis as it enters the large intestine's 1.5 m length. Food on average can take anywhere between 24 and 72 hours to digest fully. This depends on the food and the ability of the individual gut.

THE GUT TUBE

When we were forming as embryos we started off life as a series of tubes. The first tube was the neural tube which became the central nervous system. The next tube to be formed was the gut tube which became the gastrointestinal tract, the lungs, the pancreas and the liver. That is most of the organs of the body. The gut tube started simple. One long tube which almost immediately began to grow in length around the mid gut to produce the intestines. For a while the gut grew out of the lower cavity into the yolk sac, so it could find room to grow. Each part of the gut from the mouth to the rectum has developed a special gut wall that distinguishes it from the rest of the gut. However, in essence the gut is still there as one tube even though it became much more sophisticated and has division within it. Here's an exercise to come into a sense of your gut as a whole unit of function.

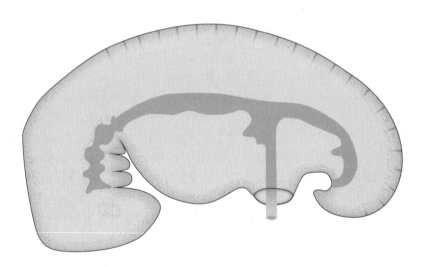

The gut tube in an embryo

Exercise: The gut as a tube

Close your eyes, relax and come into a sense of your whole body. Begin to become aware of your gut tube. Picture the early embryo and a sense of the early gut as a midline tube in the front of the body. Spend some time with this image and experience. Allow the detail of the upper part of the tube to come through. How does your mouth feel right now? Is your jaw tight, can you relax your tongue into the base of your mouth, how much saliva is there in your mouth? Form some saliva and gently swallow. Track the wave of peristalsis down your oesophagus. Can you feel the wave pass down behind your heart, into your stomach?

Become aware of the left side of your upper abdomen, underneath your heart and diaphragm. How full or empty is your stomach right now? Can you remember having a really full stomach? Can you remember feeling really hungry and wanting to fill your stomach? Move through your stomach into the duodenum. Can you visualize the C shape, the connections to the gall bladder and pancreas? Can you begin to get a sense of all the activity in this area? Take a detour into the right side under the diaphragm – feel the powerhouse of the liver. It's huge, maybe dense, fluid, warm, humming with activity. What words fit to your sense of your own liver?

Come back into the gut tube and duodenum. Move through into the metres of twists and turns in the small intestine. How does it feel around your belly button? Picture the transition into the large intestine, go up, across and down. How full is your rectum right now, how tightly squeezed is your anus?

Offer a sense of relaxation all the way from your jaw to your diaphragm and cardiac sphincter, to the exit of the stomach (the pyloric sphincter) to the ileocecal valve deep in the right iliac fossa all the way through to the anal sphincter. Can you finish with a sense of the whole gut tube and its accessory organs?

YOU ARE HOW YOU PERISTALT

How many people have digestive issues? Most people in the modern world suffer from some form of irritation of the gut lining and so can't efficiently absorb nutrition from the food they eat and therefore their metabolic energy is decreased, so they become tired and lacking in energy. The two go hand in hand. Poor digestion equals low energy. The gut's primary instinct is to peristalt. The whole length of the gut is a series of longitudinal and circular smooth muscles with an internal membrane. The muscles are wired to contract in a wave-like motion that looks just like an oscillation wave. The combination of long and circular contractions produces a wave-like rippling to allow food to pass along the length of the gut. This ability is one of the events to diminish most as the gut becomes incompetent and quickly this will lead to congestion. So then as you eat you bloat because food is not being moved along the length of the gut sufficiently well. Peristalsis is the healthy movement of the gut. One wave travels the full length of the tube in about nine seconds.

Exercise: Test your peristalsis

Hands on your abdomen. You need to have eaten an hour or so before and you should find that your gut is moving around like there's a python in there. That's the sign of a healthy gut. The movement should come in regular bouts and be smooth and coordinated. If your gut is lurching around and it's disturbing you then you have irritable bowel and your gut will be inflamed and lots of gas will be produced. If your gut is hardly moving at all then your system is really struggling to digest and the gut's competency has been reduced dramatically. Find out how you peristalt and look at what you are eating.

THE WORLD OF MUCOUS MEMBRANES

The gut is the centre of mucus production in the body. Its internal surface needs to be coated with mucus to allow food to pass through so it acts as a lubricant and the mucus protects the membranous layer of the gut. It also creates a neutral pH.

Most people think mucus is something that comes from the nose. But actually most of the mucus in the body is in the gut. Prodigious amounts of it are produced over the lifetime of the gut. The nose is just the beginning of the mucous membrane tract that flows the length of the gut and into the lungs. It keeps things neutral so that digestive enzymes don't digest the gut walls, and slimy so that food can slide down through peristalsis. When things go wrong physiologically it tends to be because the gut has become too acidic through eating food that is high in acid content. And mucus production has gone down because the gut membranes have lost their wisdom maybe through poor blood flow into the gut or equally as likely the nervous system is stressed and has confused the cells that produce mucus. So there's not enough mucus or it's too sticky so that nothing can move. The good news is that it doesn't need to be like this. You can have the best gut wall if you eat what the body likes. There's plenty of information available about the right balance of foods for good health – just go on the internet or into a book store, and there will be sections dedicated to eating wholesome and nutritious food. So for once in the history of man, no one can say that there is a lack of intelligent information. Still people are trying to poison themselves through too much sugar, salt and the wrong kinds of fat, plus overeating all of these and eating low energy foods, so that the gut becomes congested and stagnant. Your digestive fire goes out leading to constipation, bloating and highly acidic blood, then your immune system reduces in effectiveness.

STRESS AND YOUR GUT

People's lives are highly stressful. The human system was not designed to cope with such high levels of stress and it means that most people are in fight or flight mode, leading to internal physiological chaos that changes the chemical balance of the body and makes us less intelligent not only at a physical level but mentally too. So you can't think clearly any more.

For some reason when people are upset, distressed, over-whelmed or stressed they turn to fatty food, sugar and salt, and stop drinking water. Emotionally this acts to bury things. Making your system as sludgy as possible will mean you become physically desensitized which makes things more bearable. Then when you get tired you pep yourself up with sugar hits.

Here's a way of teasing yourself away from this dark de-structive spiral of behaviour:

- *Be rational.* Think intelligently about what your body needs for health and base a life on this. It's logical to eat the right food and to keep your system balanced, then you have more energy and you are happier.

- *Want to embrace life.* Wanting to live is a prime require-ment for honouring your body, and feeding it the right things and taking care of it go hand in hand with this. This means you will not want to abuse your gut; you will want to honour it with the most suitable foods for your digestion.

- *Feel your vitality.* You've forgotten what your life force feels like. Re-experiencing this is very useful and brings you back to a vibrant world. You can use the exercises in this chapter to reveal some of the intelligent life within your gut. Giving it the right attention will allow it to show you health.

Exercise: Stories in the gastrointestinal tract

Close your eyes. Be with a sense of your whole system. This is the integrated you. Now shift your perception to a sense of the whole of your digestive system from the mouth to the anus. Engage with the sense of soft, hollow, fluid, active organs in the front of your body, especially in your belly, but also connecting up to your mouth and down to your pelvis. Allow some time for your perceptions to settle; try and keep a sense of your gut tube as part of your whole body. Are there any words, phrases, images or emotions that fit to how your gut feels right now? What is your gut instinct of how you are right now? Explore your felt sense of what you are digesting and ruminating over in your gut, your body, your life. Allow the possibility that these background sensations in your gut may reflect your visceral response to the important stories in your life. Do not try and change what you are feeling. When it feels right, slowly disengage the focus on your gut, connect to the weight of your body in the chair, hear the sounds in the room and slowly open your eyes. How do you feel?

THE ABDOMINAL CAVITY

The abdominal cavity is the home of the gut and the majority of the digestive process. The organ cavities are powerful places to get a sense of and can lead to a change in your body awareness, creating an increased sense of volume and spaciousness that makes you feel more three-dimensional and substantial. Often we can be way too oriented to the surface of our bodies. There's lots of emphasis on this in the modern world – the way we look and our appearance is an obsession. Moving away from the surface to the depths of the body produces a very distinct change – a more internalized and introspective state emerges that literally brings a sense of depth to you experientially, physiologically and emotionally. Here are a couple of exercises that will help bring you into relationship with your intero-receptors which are the autonomic nervous system's sense organs spread throughout the gut and particularly in the connective tissue around the gut and the peritoneum.

Exercise: Feeling the three cavities

Follow your breath into the chest and the thoracic cavity. See if you can have a sense of the cavity space and the organs within it. Let your breathing deepen so that your abdominal wall rises and falls. This will allow you to follow your breathing into the abdominal cavity. Feel the different size and volume of the space and the different quality in the organs. It's completely different to the thoracic cavity. The abdomen is anatomically divided into the abdominal and pelvic cavities. Notice the difference between the upper abdomen and the pelvic cavity. The abdomen and the thorax are the anterior spaces of the body. Move your attention backwards into the nervous system space bounded by the vertebral column and cranium. This is another cavity, very different in shape. How is this cavity, containing the central nervous system, different? How do all three affect each other?

Exercise: The cavities and the diaphragm

The diaphragm is the partition between the upper and lower cavities of the torso and is in direct contact with almost all the organs of the body. So the health of the diaphragm has a profound effect on the health of the organs. The intention of this exercise is to bring you into an appreciation of the thoracic and abdominal cavities as spaces separated by the diaphragm. Sitting comfortably, bring your awareness to your breathing and see if you can feel

the movements of the diaphragm. As you get a deeper connection to the diaphragm, open up to the space on either side of it.
Now invite the thoracic space into your perceptual field. Notice
the size of the space and the containment of the rib cage. Then
invite the abdominal space and notice how different the space is.
Now be equally aware of both spaces coming together around the
diaphragm. Sit with this for a few minutes and note the changes
that take place.

GUT WALL/LUNG WALL

It's a pity these are described as walls. A wall is something that
keeps things out or in and really it's not just about that. It's more
about an interactive process that involves softening and yield-
ing to pressure both internal and external, so it's really more
about being a sensitive-in-discriminating membrane. The most
important places in your body are the gut wall and the bronchial sacs, as these are the interfaces where absorption (of food
and air respectively) takes place. The gut wall creates a huge
amount of surface area through structures called villi which are
small finger-like protuberances throughout the length of the
small intestine. In essence these are similar to the alveoli in the
lungs which also create huge amounts of surface area for the
diffusion of gases across the surface. Both offer a meeting place
between our blood and the outside world and both are about
taking in. In the lungs we call it breathing and in the gut we
call it digesting but in a way you are breathing food through
your gut and digesting oxygen through your lungs. It's the
same process. For the gut it's about the molecules in food dif-
fusing across the membrane of the villi into the bloodstream.
The body ideally takes what it wants and a smart gut allows
the important molecules across and into the bloodstream. Guts
with low intelligence either don't allow the right compounds to
be absorbed or don't allow enough to be absorbed. It can get

very confusing and suddenly the whole body is suffering from a lack of raw materials and the body must feel like it's starved, as if you are holding your chest tight and hardly breathing in and gasping for air. So no wonder your energy is low.

Where does your energy come from?

Your body obtains energy from:

- air through breathing
- food through digestion
- rest through sleep and relaxation.

At least a third of your entire energy comes from eating and digestion. All three are necessary for the health of the body and you will find that if one of these is not in harmony it will affect the other energy streams. So poor breathing will affect the digestion and interfere with your ability to deep sleep.

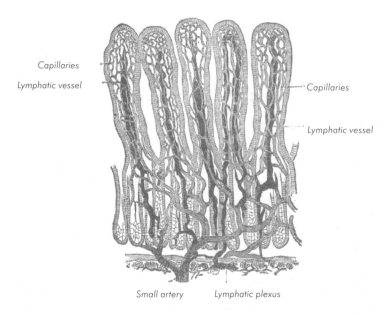

Capillaries

Lymphatic vessel

Capillaries

Lymphatic vessel

Small artery   Lymphatic plexus

Gut lining

Similarly poor digestion will affect your breathing and will definitely create unrest in your sleep. Insomnia and stress will bring all your body systems down.

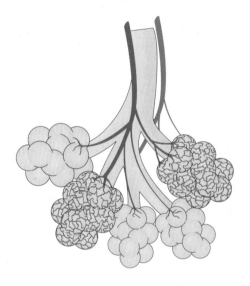

Alveoli

THE GUT IMMUNE SYSTEM

The digestive tract's immune system is essential to maintaining a bacteria free body – 70 per cent of your immune system is in your gut. The gut immune system is made up of several types of lymphoid tissue that store immune cells, such as T and B lymphocytes, that carry out attacks and defend against bacteria, viruses and toxins. The immune system in the gut starts with the tonsils and adenoids (tonsils in the pharynx), Peyer's patches in the small intestines and lymph tissue in the appendix. Commonly people have lots of these removed because of inflammation and this reduces the body's immune strength.

The largest part of the immune system in our body is in the mucosal lining in the gut. The intestines are selectively permeable to proper nutrients as the contents of the intestines pass by. Normally, only certain nutrients are absorbed if they are sufficiently broken down and in the right form. Everything else is selectively blocked out. But when the pores are too big or the screening process breaks down, the intestines become hyper-permeable. Leaky gut syndrome is a term used when the intestines become damaged, more openings develop in the gut wall, and the wall becomes more 'porous' to the extent that some of the contents passing through the intestines are allowed to get into the bloodstream when they should be kept out.

Not just food particles slip through. Pathogens, toxins and other types of 'waste' get through that should normally be screened out. Insufficiently broken down food particles or toxins may cause the liver to work much harder trying to clean everything out. The liver may not be able to keep up with all the detoxification demands sent its way and the toxin load starts building up in the body. When this happens, the immune system kicks into gear. If not removed right away, the toxins can migrate through the body and settle in any of the different tissues they pass by. This leads to inflammation in whatever part of the body they settle in.

Now inflammation is the major difficulty for the body. This puts even more pressure on the immune system to cover even more ground in defending the body. With the immune system running on 'high' on a regular basis, it may be spread thinly over a wide area, defending the gut, cleaning the blood, fighting inflammation, warding off pathogens, and so on. Many autoimmune conditions start this way.

THE LIVER IS THE BLOOD PORTAL

The guardian of the whole body is the liver. It's the inspector and the gatekeeper for the relationship between the gut and the rest of the body. It makes decisions about what enters the bloodstream from the intestines and constantly filters the blood and removes worn out cells. Food gets broken down in the stomach and duodenum and starts to be absorbed through the small intestines into a special blood network connected to the liver called the hepatic portal system (hepatic means liver). When the blood comes to the liver it slows down as it passes through lots of hexagonal shaped structures (hepatocytes) that allow the liver cells to interact with the blood in order to filter and sort it. That's why the liver is so hot – it's a factory of activity and its cells need a lot of energy to drive the many processes

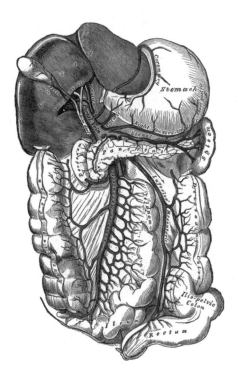

The portal system

that take place within it. It's also a very big organ and occupies a large section of the abdominal cavity. Typically it weighs up to 3 kg and it is full of blood – up to a pint at any time. It is one of the blood reservoirs of the body.

Why is the liver the greatest organ in the universe?

The liver is the largest and most complex organ in the body. It cleanses 600 litres of blood daily, processing all matter, food or otherwise, that finds itself in the system. All toxic material ingested through the portal vein system (via the stomach and intestines) will be acted upon by the liver and neutralized, preventing absorption into the main bloodstream. This includes chemicals, preservatives, nicotine, alcohol, artificial substances, etc.

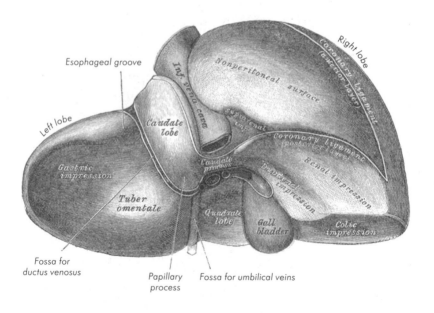

The liver

Chemically the liver plays host to over 500 different kinds of chemical processes! Some of these processes involve breaking down complex chemicals; others involve synthesis, especially of protein molecules, as well as deactivating drugs and hormones.

- Proteins are involved in structural strength, muscle contraction, regulation, buffering, clotting, transport, ion channels, receptors and the immune system (most things in the body), which makes the liver a very critical organ in the maintenance of healthy body function.

- Unwanted proteins are broken down to their amino acids (depending on current body requirements), and then reassembled into the correct sequence to create new proteins required at that time.

- The liver deals with nutrients arriving from the intestine, for example, converting glucose to glycogen and storing it (carbohydrate metabolism). The liver stores a fifth of the body's supply of glycogen!

- Special cells that line the liver's blood vessels mop up unwanted elements and infectious organisms, removing them from the gut.

- The liver greatly aids the immune system by creating specialized 'complement' proteins which are sensitive to specific foreign substances. Complement proteins are activated by and work with antibodies. They cause lysing (bursting) of target cells and signal to phagocytes that a cell needs to be removed. A phagocyte is a type of white blood cell that can engulf and destroy foreign organisms, cells and particles.

- Toxic substances like alcohol in the bloodstream are converted to harmless waste products. Ammonia is removed by turning it into urea.

- Hormones are removed from the bloodstream by the liver so they don't continue to activate the body after their job is done. This is why it takes time to wind down after the sympathetic system activates hormone releases.

- Digestive lipid products arrive at the liver, some of which are used to generate vital fatty substances, mainly cholesterol which is an essential ingredient in some hormone construction and in nerve function.

The liver receives both oxygen-rich arterial blood from the hepatic artery, plus venous blood from the hepatic portal vein which is rich in nutrients from the digestive viscera. The filtered and processed blood exits the liver via the central vein. The liver's hepatocyte cells can produce bile which is stored mainly in the gall bladder. Bile is an alkaline solution containing bile salts, bile pigments, cholesterol, triglycerides, phospholipids and electrolytes (magnesium/calcium and potassium/sodium). Bile emulsifies fats in the intestines, and can also absorb fat-soluble vitamins, mainly A, D, E and K, which are important for night vision, normal skin integrity, nerve function and normal blood clotting.

The bile salts that the liver generates are recycled and reused by the liver via the small intestine (ileum) extracting them back into the blood and returning them to the liver.

Interestingly in Chinese medicine the liver is considered to be the organ that creates balance and harmony for all the other organs and this is just what it does through cleaning and purifying the blood.

Exercise: Decongesting your liver

Often the liver becomes congested and sluggish in its action and purging or detoxification of the liver is vital to regain health. Here are a couple of easy ways to bring this about without swallowing lots of supplements or fasting. First bring your hands to your liver. It occupies the whole of the middle right of your torso and lies under your diaphragm surrounded by the rib cage. The left lobe of the liver runs across the solar plexus. So put one hand over the solar plexus and the other on the lower right side of the rib cage. Now follow your breathing and come into the sensations of the air moving into your lungs. Stay with this for a while and imagine that your breath can move deeper through the diaphragm and into the body of the liver. So now as you breathe in you are breathing into your liver as well as your lungs. The liver will feel different from doing this. Sometimes it can become hot or achy or strained before it starts to get heavier and more relaxed and then there is a sense of it expanding, so that your breath feels like it's moving into a much bigger space.

Another useful exercise is to put your hands on your liver as above and shake your liver by bringing your body into a bouncing movement. Flex around your knees so that your body drops and then straighten your knees so it rises and continue letting the body rise and fall. Let the rising and falling pivot around the liver under your hands. Be gentle about it at first. This will feel like the liver is gently oscillating. Continue this for several minutes and as your body warms up the liver will feel like it's getting heavier and all parts of it are joining in the movement and freeing up. Let your body move how it wants now. The movements may become much stronger and subtly change in frequency and quality to produce a variety of movements.

THE PANCREAS – THE HIDDEN ORGAN

This is an interesting organ. It's the deepest organ in the body and lies right at the centre of the torso. Most of us just don't know the pancreas is there as it's so hidden. Ask people where their kidneys are or their liver or heart, guts or lungs and they will know with reasonable accuracy and probably have some sense of the organ within them, but ask them where the pancreas is and that might get blank stares. It's not an organ of conversation. The only people to talk about the pancreas are people who are ill with a pancreatic condition or anatomists. This is a vital organ that carries out many key functions of the body and is a cross between a digestive organ and an endocrine gland. One part of it manufactures digestive enzymes for breaking down of food after it leaves the stomach and the other part produces vital hormones, the best known being insulin. If the pancreas becomes inflamed or irritated this can be a life threatening event.

Exercise: Pancreas as centre of the body

With one hand over the area of the stomach and the other hand on the back of the body mirroring the front hand, you are in contact with essential elements from all the major systems of the body. This contact will put you in touch with the spine, postural muscles, the lymphatic system, the end of the spinal cord, many important autonomic centres, major endocrine glands and nearly all the major organs. This is a very packed area of the body and very busy. At the centre of all of this busy part of the body lies the pancreas, underneath the stomach. It's a long spongy yellow organ lying across the body from the spleen to the duodenum. Think of a long yellow cylinder-shaped organ between your hands and you may get a sense of it deep towards the back wall of the cavity. Stay with the pancreas as the centre of your body and see what happens.

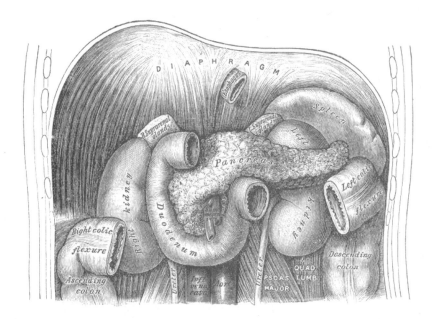

The pancreas

INSTINCT AND YOUR PERITONEUM

The guts are wrapped in a connective tissue bag called the peritoneum which is one whole structure. It both wraps each of the organs and surrounds all of them. The small intestine is wrapped in a special tissue called the mesentery. It's a loose connective tissue layer that supports the nerve and blood supply and holds the intestines in place within the abdominal cavity. The transverse colon, which is draped across the abdomen, also has a special mesentery wrap that holds it in place. In the front of both of these is a special part of the peritoneum called the greater omentum – a large connective tissue shaped like an apron hanging from the stomach.

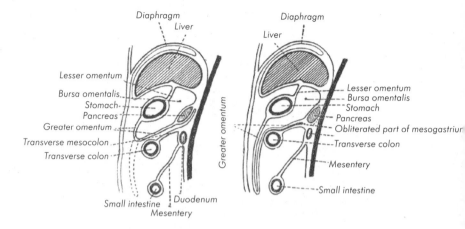

The peritoneum

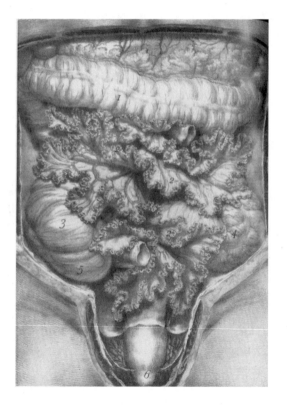

The gastrointestinal tract

Exercise: Your peritoneum is a sensory organ

Bring your awareness to your abdominal wall. This is a mix of skin and muscles. Let your attention sink into them. When you do this, feel your muscles engage slightly in response. Let your attention deepen so that you shift out of the wall and into the cavity. This should feel instantly like entering a large cavernous space. The first thing you come into contact with is the outer layer of the peritoneum. This is adjacent to the underside of the abdominal muscles. It feels light and delicate and defines a whole separate space surrounded by this membrane. See if you can get a sense of this. When you do it feels like you have an internal balloon that rises up to your diaphragm and down into the pelvis. If you deepen down again you will come into the viscera contained within the peritoneum. This is mostly the gut but also the liver and pancreas. If you get interested in the gut you will quickly feel the length of a tube that is bound by part of the peritoneum called the mesentery. If your guts fell out of your abdomen the mesentery would look like a big fan shape angling back into the centre of the body. All these different parts of the peritoneum provide lots of information to the brain about the position of the organs and the state of the blood supply and immune system. They also have an ability to pick up on all kinds of information from outside the body. Notice how your peritoneum responds next time you stand next to someone, especially someone you don't know. There is commonly a reaction and perhaps this is part of the response we call gut instinct.

GUT BRAIN

New science is showing that we can talk of a heart brain and a belly brain. The nervous connections around the heart (thoracic ganglia and its intrinsic nervous system) have their own independent circuits. Similarly the enteric nervous system, coordinating gut activity, has its own independent processing outside the central nervous system. Just look at the way the small intestine looks like the folds of the cerebral brain.

The enteric nervous system is capable of autonomous functions such as the coordination of reflexes, but it is fundamentally part of the autonomic nervous system and is powerfully affected by stress and emotional states. It has as many as 100 million neurons, one thousandth of the number of neurons in the brain, and considerably more than the number of neurons in the spinal cord. So after the brain it is the most complex part of the nervous system.

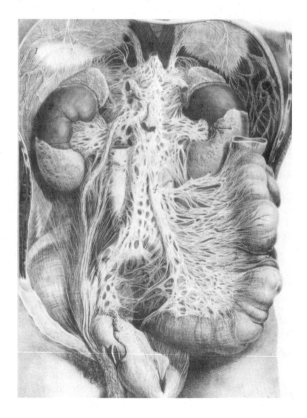

Enteric nervous system

The enteric nervous system has been described as a 'second brain'. There are several reasons for this. The enteric nervous system can operate autonomously. It normally communicates with the central nervous system through the parasympathetic (e.g. via the vagus nerve) and sympathetic (e.g. via the pre-vertebral ganglia) nervous systems. However, vertebrate studies show that when the vagus nerve is severed, the enteric nervous system continues to function.

In vertebrates the enteric nervous system includes motor and sensory neurons and interneurons, all of which make the enteric nervous system capable of carrying reflexes and acting as an integrating centre in the absence of central nervous system input. The sensory neurons report on mechanical and chemical conditions. Through intestinal muscles, the motor neurons control peristalsis and churning of intestinal contents. Other neurons control the secretion of enzymes. The enteric nervous system also makes use of more than 30 neurotransmitters, most of which are identical to the ones found in the central nervous system, such as acetylcholine, dopamine and serotonin. The enteric nervous system has the capacity to alter its response depending on such factors as bulk and nutrient composition. In addition, the enteric nervous system contains support cells which are similar to astroglia of the brain and a diffusion barrier around the capillaries surrounding ganglia which is similar to the blood–brain barrier of cerebral blood vessels.

Exercise: Being in your gut

Part of our gut instinct and gut response to events and people comes from using our gut brain. How instinctive you are depends on how well you can operate from this brain by getting out of your head. Many emotional and instinctual responses take place here that are not part of thinking or analysing the way the cerebral brain does. Next time you have a decision to make or are unsure about a course of action or relationships, try shifting out of your head into your gut and instinctualizing the situation. You can do this by practising being in your gut. The next time you have a difficult decision to make, first try putting your hands on your abdomen while standing, one hand in the small of the back and the other on your gut. From this position move your pelvis in a circle keeping your hands in place. Stay with this for a few minutes then circle in the opposite direction. Now keeping your hands in place stay still for a couple of minutes. Now try thinking about the decision you need to make and see what comes to you. You've stimulated your enteric nervous system and the separate and unique intelligence of this system will offer a different perspective and a new way to understand.

About the Author

Ged Sumner is a practising craniosacral therapist and Chi Kung teacher. He has also studied shiatsu, healing and attachment-based psychoanalytical psychotherapy. He has taught biodynamic craniosacral therapy as a senior tutor and course director for the Craniosacral 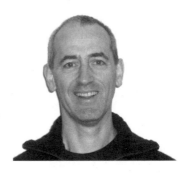 Therapy Educational Trust's (CTET) practitioner trainings in London and as a senior tutor for Resonance Trainings courses in Australia and New Zealand. He set up the Fountain Clinic in London which is a specialized Craniosacral Therapy Clinic (www.fountainclinic.com). He also set up and directed a 'Living Anatomy' training for CTET offering a holistic view of the body's anatomy and physiology. He is a director of the Healthy Living Centre (www.thehealthylivingcentre.co.uk), a multi-disciplinary alternative therapy practice in London. He is also director of the College of Chi Kung offering classes, workshops, retreats and a Chi Kung Teacher Training programme in London and Australia (www.elementalchikung.com). He has a degree in chemistry and currently lives in Australia with his partner and has three children.

Index

brain *cont.*
  understanding of 122–3
  and white and grey matter 145–51
brain stem 129–30, 176–8
breathing
  and body health 47–9, 54–5
  and the diaphragm 49–51
  exercises 51–2, 55–7
  function of 47
  importance of 62
  and posture 53–4

calcium 31–2
cerebellum 128–9, 130
cerebrospinal fluid 119
cerebrum 127–8
Chi Kung 8
Circle of Willis 185, 186
collagen 20–1
coronary artery 104
cortisol 171–2
cranium 28–30

Descartes, Rene 122
diaphragm
  description of 49–51
  and emotions 57–8
  exercises 51–2, 59
  function of 57
  health of 51
  and nature 59
  and relationships 58
dura mater 125

eating
  and the abdominal cavity 199–201
  and the digestive process 191–3
  exercises 195, 196
  and the gut tube 194–5
  and mucus membranes 197
  and peristalsis 196
emotions
  and the body 181–3
  and the brain 178–80
  exercises 180–1, 182–3, 189–90

and the heart 168–70
and stress 186–90
exercises
  and adrenal exhaustion 174–5
  and the automatic nervous system 159–60, 166
  and blood 101, 108–9
  and the body 182–3
  and bones 22–3, 32–3
  and the brain 119–21, 126, 133, 146–8, 177–8, 185
  and breathing 51–2, 55–7
  and the diaphragm 51–2, 59
  and digestion 195, 196
  and the emotions 180–1, 182–3, 189–90
  and the face 28–9
  and the feet 95–7
  and the gut 195, 196, 199, 200–1, 213, 215–16
  and the head 29–30
  and the heart 101, 169–70
  and the jaw 78–80
  and the joints 67–8, 70, 71–2
  and the liver 209
  and the lungs 59–60
  and the nervous system 137–8, 143
  and neurons 143
  and the pancreas 210
  place for 14
  and posture 55–6, 70
  and the ribs 61
  and the spine 40, 42, 43, 70, 71–2, 88, 90
  and walking 86, 88, 90, 92, 94, 95–7
  and white and grey matter 146–8
eye sockets 27–8

face
  bones in 25–8
  exercises 28–9
falx 124
feet 95–7
fibrous joint 64
Freud, Sigmund 8, 9